CRASH COURSE

Gastroenterology

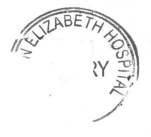

CRASH COURSE

Third Edition

Gastroenterology

Series editor

Daniel Horton-Szar
BSc(Hons) MBBS(Hons) MRCGP

Northgate Medical Practice,
Canterbury,
Kent, UK

Faculty advisor

Martin Lombard
MD MSc FRCPI FRCP(Lond)

Consultant Physician and
Gastroenterologist,
Royal Liverpool University
Hospital and
Senior Lecturer in Medicine,
University of Liverpool,
Liverpool, UK

Paul Collins
MBBCh MRCP

Lecturer in Medicine, School of Clinical Science, University
of Liverpool, and Honorary Registrar in Gastroenterology,
Royal Liverpool University Hospital, Liverpool, UK

First and second edition authors:

Emma Lam

Martin Lombard

Christopher Fox

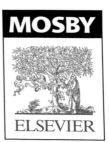

MOSBY

ELSEVIER

Edinburgh • London • New York • Oxford • Philadelphia • St Louis • Sydney • Toronto 2008

MOSBY
ELSEVIER

Commissioning Editor	Alison Taylor
Development Editor	Ailsa Laing
Project Manager	Gail Wright
Page Design	Sarah Russell
Icon Illustrations	Geo Parkin
Cover Design	Stewart Larking
Illustration Management	Merlyn Harvey

First edition 1999
Second edition 2004
Third edition 2008

ISBN 978-0-7234-3470-2

British Library Cataloguing in Publication Data
A catalogue record for this book is available from the British Library

Library of Congress Cataloging in Publication Data
A catalog record for this book is available from the Library of Congress

Notice
Knowledge and best practice in this field are constantly changing. As new research and experience
broaden our knowledge, changes in practice, treatment and drug therapy may become necessary or
appropriate. Readers are advised to check the most current information provided (i) on procedures
featured or (ii) by the manufacturer of each product to be administered, to verify the recommended
dose or formula, the method and duration of administration, and contraindications. It is the
responsibility of the practitioner, relying on their own experience and knowledge of the patient, to
make diagnoses, to determine dosages and the best treatment for each individual patient, and to
take all appropriate safety precautions. To the fullest extent of the law, neither the Publisher nor the
Authors assumes any liability for any injury and/or damage to persons or property arising out of or
related to any use of the material contained in this book.

The Publisher

The approach of medical exams and the first clinical job can be an overwhelming experience. Whether you are approaching the subject for the first time, or are seeking a comprehensive revision tool, this book will provide the facts in a clear, concise and accessible way.

I hope that you enjoy using this book and that it helps instill confidence and ease the transition from exams to wards.

Paul Collins

Having recently negotiated the daunting hurdles of medical finals and MRCP, I can certainly appreciate the value of a book such as this. The logical structure and friendly format provides enough detail for a distinction student, whilst simultaneously serving as a concise revision text.

I hope that, in addition to facilitating success with your undergraduate exams, it will also aid the transition to pre-registration house officer, and assist with the various gastrointestinal problems that you will undoubtedly face.

There is light at the end of the tunnel. This book will help prevent you becoming lost along the way!

Christopher Fox

Despite their best intentions and notice of timetables, all students find that exams come too soon. *Crash Course* is written by people who've been there for people who are getting there! The clinical series is largely written by young doctors in training who have recently passed their exams and who know what you need to know to pass and excel in your exam. This book on gastroenterology tells you that, but I hope it is comprehensive enough to give you even more—a good grounding in gastroenterology. It may therefore prove useful as a brief reference for forgotten facts even for those not doing exams. It doesn't pretend to give all of the detail required to practice gastroenterology, but should be used as a primer for those starting out in a career in gastroenterology and as a crash course for those coming up to examinations. The illustrations in this book pack in thousands more words than we could in the text and I hope you will enjoy learning from them.

More than a decade has now passed since work began on the first editions of the *Crash Course* series, and over 4 years since the publication of the second editions. The involvement of a new author with each successive edition has ensured that the text remains fresh. Facts relating to clinical practice have been kept up to date and abreast of current developments in the field. The style and layout has been refined successively to a very high specification. You will not find as much comprehensive information crammed into such a small space in such an understandable way in any other text. If you follow the text and self-examination exercises, you should excel in any test in gastroenterology.

Martin Lombard
Faculty Advisor

Medicine never stands still, and the work of keeping this series relevant for today's students is an ongoing process. These third editions build upon the success of the preceding books and incorporate a great deal of new and revised material, keeping the series up to date with the latest medical research and developments in pharmacology and current best practice.

As always, we listen to feedback from the thousands of students who use *Crash Course* and have made further improvements to the layout and structure of the books. Each chapter now starts with a set of learning objectives, and the self-assessment sections have been enhanced and brought up to date with modern exam formats. We have also worked to integrate material on communication skills and gems of clinical wisdom from practising doctors. This will not only add to the interest of the text but will reinforce the principles being described.

Despite fully revising the books, we hold fast to the principles on which we first developed the series: *Crash Course* will always bring you all the information you need to revise in compact, manageable volumes that integrate pathology and therapeutics with best clinical practice. The books still maintain the balance between clarity and conciseness, and provide sufficient depth for those aiming at distinction. The authors are junior doctors who have recent experience of the exams you are now facing, and the accuracy of the material is checked by senior clinicians and faculty members from across the UK.

I wish you all the best for your future careers!

Dr Dan Horton-Szar
Series Editor

Acknowledgements

Grateful thanks to the following at Royal Liverpool University Hospital for their helpful contributions and comments to this book: Dr Conall Garvey, Consultant Radiologist for all of the radiology pictures; Dr Fiona Campbell, Consultant Pathologist for all of the histology photomicrographs; and Tracy Norris for the graphs of oesophageal manometry and pH. We would also like to thank our mentors and students, respectively, for all that they have taught us and Emma Lam, the author of the first edition of *Crash Course: Gastroenterology*.

Dedication

For our families

Contents

Contents

Part IV: Self-assessment 223

Glossary

Achalasia Motility disorder of the oesophagus characterized by a failure of the lower oesophageal sphincter to relax after swallowing.

ALD Alcoholic liver disease.

ALT Alanine aminotransferase.

AMA Antimitochondrial antibody.

ANA Anti-nuclear antibody.

ANCA Anti-neutrophil cytoplasmic antibody.

Anorexia Symptom of decreased appetite.

Antiemetic Drug used to prevent vomiting.

Anti-LKM antibody Anti-liver kidney microsomal antibody.

Anti-SMA antibody Anti-smooth muscle antibody.

Antispasmodic Drug used to reduce muscle contraction. Used in irritable bowel syndrome to reduce gastrointestinal motility.

APC Adenomatosis polyposis coli-a-tumour suppressor gene.

ARDS Adult respiratory distress syndrome.

Ascites Excess fluid in the peritoneal cavity.

AST Aspartate aminotransferase.

Barrett's oesophagus Premalignant condition characterized by a change in the mucosal lining of the distal oesophagus from squamous to columnar. Associated with gastro-oesophageal reflux.

Biliary atresia Congenital absence of the bile duct.

BSP Bromsulphthalein.

CBD Common bile duct.

CD Crohn's disease.

Cholestasis Failure of bile to flow.

CMV Cytomegalovirus.

Colitis Inflammation of the colon.

COPD Chronic obstructive pulmonary disease.

CRC Colorectal cancer.

CSF Cerebrospinal fluid.

CT Computed tomography.

DEXA Dual energy X-ray absorptiometry.

DIC Disseminated intravascular coagulation.

Diverticulitis Subserosal inflammation associated with diverticulosis.

Diverticulosis Presence of outpouching of the mucosa and submucosa through points of weakness in the muscle layer of the colonic wall.

DU Duodenal ulcer.

Dyspepsia Generic term used to describe symptoms of indigestion. It encompasses symptoms of heartburn, early satiety, upper abdominal discomfort, flatulence, hiccups and belching.

Dysphagia Difficulty swallowing.

Dysplasia Abnormality of cell maturation within a tissue. It is premalignant.

EATL Enteropathy-associated T lymphoma.

EBV Epstein-Barr virus.

ELISA Enzyme-linked immunosorbent assay.

EN Enteral nutrition.

Endoscopy Examination of a body cavity using a flexible optical instrument.

ERCP Endoscopic retrograde cholangiopancreatography.

EUS Endoscopic ultrasound.

FAP Familial adenomatous polyposis.

FBC Full blood count.

FOB Faecal occult blood.

Fundoplication A surgical procedure used to treat GORD. The fundus (upper part) of the stomach is plicated (wrapped) around the lower oesophagus.

GGT Gamma-glutamyl transferase.

GORD Gastro-oesophageal reflux disease.

GU Gastric ulcer.

Haematemesis Vomiting of blood.

Haematochezia Passage of blood per rectum.

HAV Hepatitis A virus.

HBV Hepatitis B virus.

HCC Hepatocellular carcinoma.

HCV Hepatitis C virus.

Hepatic encephalopathy Altered behaviour and neurology occurring in advanced liver disease as a consequence of toxic metabolites passing across the blood-brain barrier.

Hepatitis Inflammation of the liver.

HIDA Hydroxy imino-diacetic acid.

HLA Human leukocyte antigen.

HNPCC Hereditary non-polyposis colorectal cancer.

HUS Haemolytic uraemic syndrome.

IBD Inflammatory bowel disease.

IBS Irritable bowel syndrome.

IDA Imino-iodoacetic acid.

IEL Intraepithelial lymphocytes.

INR International normalized ratio.

Laparoscopy Surgical procedure in which a flexible optical instrument is introduced into the body through an incision.

LDH Lactate dehydrogenase.

LOS Lower oesophageal sphincter.

MALT Mucosa-associated lymphoid tissue.

Melaena Passage of digested blood per rectum signifying blood loss from the upper gastrointestinal tract.

MCV Mean cell volume.

MEN Multiple endocrine neoplasia.

MIBG Metaiodobenzylguanidine.

MRCP Magnetic resonance cholangiopancreatography.

MRI Magnetic resonance imaging.

OGD Oesophagogastroduodenoscopy.

PABA Para-aminobenzoic acid.

pANCA Perinuclear anti-neutrophil cytoplasmic antibody.

PBC Primary biliary cirrhosis.

PCR Polymerase chain reaction.

PEG Percutaneous endoscopic gastrostomy.

PET Positron emission tomography.

PPI Proton pump inhibitor.

PSC Primary sclerosing cholangitis.

Pyloroplasty Reconstruction of the distal outlet of the stomach. Usually the widening of the pylorus in cases of peptic stricturing.

SBP Spontaneous bacterial peritonitis.

SLE Systemic lupus erythematosus.

SMA Superior mesenteric artery.

TIBC Total iron-binding capacity.

TIPS Transjugular intra-hepatic portosystemic shunt.

TNM Tumour-node metastasis.

TPN Total parenteral nutrition.

UC Ulcerative colitis.

VIP Vasoactive intestinal peptide.

Waterbrash A symptom that may accompany heartburn in which the mouth floods with clear salty fluid.

THE PATIENT PRESENTS WITH ...

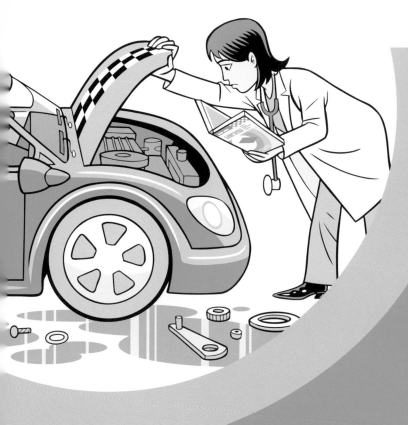

'Indigestion' encompasses a vast number of symptoms representing upper digestive tract problems with which a patient may present. These include:

- Heartburn.
- Fullness.
- Early satiety.
- Upper abdominal pain or ache.
- Flatulence.
- Hiccups.
- Belching.

The generic term that is useful to describe this constellation of symptoms is dyspepsia.

Dyspepsia:

- Is very common and occurs in up to 10% of the adult population. At least half of these 10% seek advice from their family doctor.
- Accounts for 40% of referrals to gastroenterology clinics.

Dysphagia, or difficulty in swallowing, is dealt with separately (see Ch. 2).

HISTORY OF THE PATIENT WITH INDIGESTION

When taking a history from a patient with dyspepsia, it is useful to classify the problem according to the group of symptoms present. This may be helpful in planning treatment. Dyspepsia is characterized as:

- 'Reflux-like', if heartburn or chest pain predominate.

- 'Ulcer-like', if the characteristics convey the impression of peptic ulcer disease.

'Non-ulcer dyspepsia' or 'functional dyspepsia' describes similar symptoms occurring in the absence of easily identifiable organic disease.

History of heartburn

Heartburn is the key to differentiating reflux-like dyspepsia from other forms. It is described as a burning sensation which the patient locates retrosternally (behind the sternum). It is a diffuse and poorly localized sensation, typically worse on lying and leaning forward.

A long history of heartburn followed by difficulty in swallowing (dysphagia), but improvement in the heartburn, may herald a fibrotic stricture in the lower oesophagus.

Excess saliva

'Waterbrash' is a specific phenomenon which the patient will describe as a flood of saliva in the mouth. Excess saliva is produced in the mouth and pharynx as a reflex response to acid in the lower oesophagus.

Chest pain

This is a common feature of gastro-oesophageal reflux or oesophageal spasm.

Pain due to heartburn often radiates between the shoulder blades. Oesophageal spasm (which can itself be triggered by acid reflux) more commonly causes chest pain, which occurs after a meal but can arise spontaneously. The pain is:

- Typically felt behind the sternum.
- Often severe.
- Sometimes described as 'something squeezing my inside'.

It can be difficult to distinguish oesophageal pain from cardiac chest pain. The following features of the history may help to distinguish the two:

- Oesophageal pain tends not to be provoked by exertion.
- Discomfort from oesophageal reflux can be positional, i.e. worse on lying down or stooping forward.

Some features can occur in both oesophageal and cardiac pain:

- Relief of pain by nitrates.
- Radiation of pain to the jaw or left arm.

Nausea and vomiting can accompany myocardial infarction and severe oesophageal reflux.

Nocturnal cough/asthma

Some patients with severe acid reflux do not complain of heartburn or chest pain, but develop cough or wheeze during the night when they are lying flat. They often lack symptoms during the daytime. Characteristically, they will demonstrate a 'morning dip' in their peak-flow recordings (Fig. 1.1). The bronchospasm is thought to be due to microaspiration of acid, but a vagal reflex may also be involved because, experimentally, oesophageal acid-induced bronchospasm is ablated by vagotomy.

Asthmatics have a higher than average prevalence of heartburn. Increased intra-abdominal pressure may play a role, but some drugs such as theophylline reduce the lower oesophageal sphincter tone.

Aggravating and risk factors for reflux

The most important risk factor is increased intra-abdominal pressure (Fig. 1.2) which can 'squeeze' the stomach contents upwards and, ultimately, squeeze the stomach itself through the hiatus in the diaphragm (hiatus hernia).

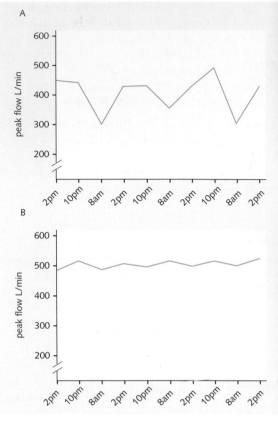

Fig. 1.1 (A) Peak flow measurement in an asthmatic demonstrating 'morning dip' due to acid reflux. (B) This was ablated when the patient took antisecretory medication before going to bed.

Fig. 1.2 Risk factors for gastro-oesophageal reflux

increased intra-abdominal pressures
- sport, e.g. weight lifting
- occupation, e.g. stooping
- asthma
- obesity
- pregnancy
drugs
- alcohol
- cigarette smoking
- caffeine
- anticholinergics

Ask about lifestyle habits and medication, as:

- Stooping and bending (occupation or sport) aggravate the problem.
- Spicy foods, or those with a high fat content, often aggravate the problem.
- Alcohol ingestion can result in increased acid secretion, delayed gastric emptying and gastritis.

- Cigarettes often make reflux symptoms worse: nicotine causes smooth muscle relaxation in the lower oesophageal sphincter.
- Caffeine and theophylline cause relaxation of the lower oesophageal sphincter.
- Those drugs with an anticholinergic action can also lower oesophageal tone (e.g. neuroleptics).

For most patients, antacids will provide some form of relief and are readily available as an over-the-counter medication.

All of these dyspeptic symptoms constitute 'gastro-oesophageal reflux disease' (GORD).

Ulcer-like dyspepsia

Epigastric pain is not a feature of GORD, but characterizes dyspepsia as 'ulcer-like'. It is a very common presenting complaint.

In patients with ulcer-like dyspepsia:

- The history is often vague.
- Sometimes patients have difficulty ascribing the term 'pain' to what they feel. The pain is often described as 'gnawing' or a persistent dull ache.

Pain due to:

- Peptic ulcer disease is occasionally more easily localized. The patient may point to a spot with one finger, although this is not a reliable sign.
- A gastric ulcer is often worse immediately after eating.

Duodenal ulcer pain is:

- Commonly relieved by antacids.
- Worse at night, or in the fasted state, so the patient will often eat or drink before going to bed at night.

Features of the history associated with peptic ulcer disease include:

- A positive family history of peptic ulcer disease.
- Smoking and alcohol consumption.
- Non-steroidal anti-inflammatory drug (NSAID) use. Ingestion can interfere with prostaglandin-mediated gastric cytoprotection.

Peptic ulcers associated with NSAID use are often painless and may present with occult bleeding.

Non-ulcer dyspepsia

'Non-ulcer dyspepsia' or 'functional dyspepsia' are terms used interchangeably for symptoms of dyspepsia that occur in the absence of demonstrable acid reflux or *Helicobacter*-related disease (duodenal and gastric ulcer; duodenitis and gastritis).

Non-ulcer dyspepsia and peptic ulcer pain can be difficult to differentiate from other causes of acute and chronic abdominal pain (see Chs 3 and 4).

EXAMINING THE PATIENT WITH INDIGESTION

Physical examination is usually unrevealing in the patient with reflux disease or oesophageal spasm.

Check for:

- Obesity or pregnancy—these may support a diagnosis of GORD.
- Chronic gastrointestinal (GI) blood loss and signs of iron deficiency—these may be caused by ulceration of the oesophageal mucosa and may indicate chronic severe acid reflux, or alternative GI pathology.
- Tooth erosion by acid—this may be a sign of very severe reflux.

Cardiac pain can sometimes be very difficult to differentiate from the pain of GORD and associated spasm. Features that may predispose to ischaemic heart disease should be looked for, such as:

- Tar staining on the fingers.
- Obesity.
- Stigmata of hypercholesterolaemia, such as xanthomas.

Tenderness on deep palpation may indicate that the patient has 'ulcer-like' dyspepsia due to gastritis or ulcer disease. Careful examination is important to exclude other causes of abdominal pain.

INVESTIGATING INDIGESTION

An algorithm for the investigation of the patient with indigestion is shown in Fig. 1.3.

In the majority of cases of reflux, the symptoms are mild and the diagnosis can often be made

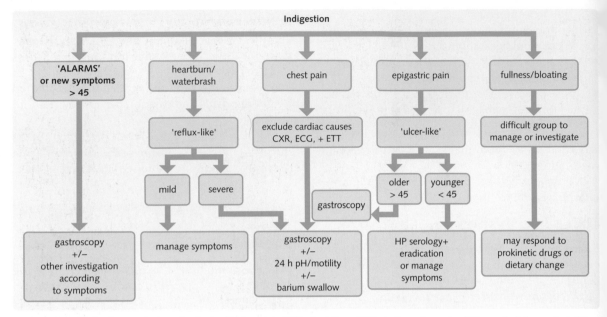

Indigestion

| 'ALARMS' or new symptoms > 45 | heartburn/ waterbrash | chest pain | epigastric pain | fullness/bloating |

'reflux-like' → exclude cardiac causes CXR, ECG, + ETT → 'ulcer-like' → difficult group to manage or investigate

mild | severe | gastroscopy | older > 45 | younger < 45

gastroscopy +/– other investigation according to symptoms | manage symptoms | gastroscopy +/– 24 h pH/motility +/– barium swallow | HP serology+ eradication or manage symptoms | may respond to prokinetic drugs or dietary change

Fig. 1.3 Algorithm for the investigation of patients with dyspepsia. (CXR, chest X-ray; ECG, electrocardiography; ETT, exercise tolerance test; HP, *Helicobacter pylori*.)

clinically and appropriate treatment commenced. More symptomatic cases may require investigation to exclude or confirm underlying oesophagitis.

In patients with indigestion, urgent referral for investigation to exclude upper GI malignancy is triggered by the 'ALARMS' symptoms.

ALARMS symptoms in dyspepsia:
- **A**naemia
- **L**oss of weight
- **A**norexia or vomiting
- **R**efractory to antisecretory medication
- **M**elaena
- **S**wallowing problems

Patients over 45 years of age with recent onset, persisting, dyspeptic symptoms should usually undergo prompt endoscopy (upper GI cancer is exceptionally rare under the age of 45 years except in familial cancer syndromes).

Investigations to consider are discussed below.

Full blood count

A full blood count may be performed to exclude underlying anaemia. A microcytic anaemia of iron deficiency can occur due to occult blood loss from oesophagitis, peptic ulceration or upper GI cancer (see Ch. 11). A high platelet count can indicate chronic GI bleeding.

Plummer–Vinson syndrome comprises iron deficiency anaemia associated with an oesophageal web and dysphagia.

Electrocardiography

Electrocardiography is particularly useful for patients with atypical sounding pain that may be due to oesophageal spasm or angina pectoris. However, non-specific T-wave changes can occur with reflux. An exercise tolerance test may be necessary to differentiate between oesophageal and cardiac pain.

Occasionally, other investigations such as a thallium scan and coronary angiography are necessary to discriminate between cardiac and oesophageal symptoms.

Chest X-ray

A chest X-ray may demonstrate a hiatus hernia behind the cardiac shadow (Fig. 1.4).

Barium swallow

Barium swallow or scintigraphy can demonstrate gastro-oesophageal reflux. In oesophageal spasm, it

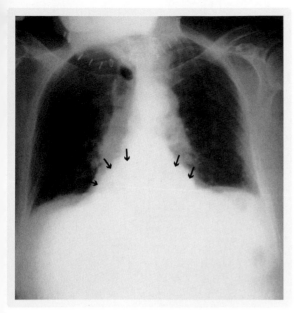

Fig. 1.4 Chest X-ray showing a hiatus hernia behind the cardiac shadow. (Incidentally shown on this X-ray are surgical staples around the neck following operative dissection.)

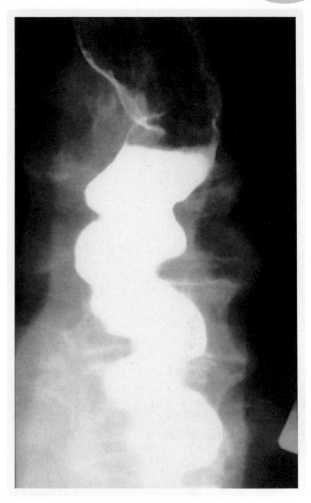

Fig. 1.5 Barium swallow demonstration of 'corkscrew' oesophagus caused by oesophageal spasm.

can give rise to a 'corkscrew' appearance, and this is usually diagnostic (Fig. 1.5).

Oesophageal manometry

This may be required to demonstrate the diffuse contraction and reduced peristalsis during a provoked attack of oesophageal spasm. Pressures in the oesophagus can be exceedingly high, and the term 'nutcracker oesophagus' has been coined for these cases.

pH monitoring

pH monitoring is usually reserved for patients with symptoms of gastro-oesophageal reflux whose symptoms are more marked than expected from the endoscopic findings and fail to respond to conventional acid suppression.

Testing for *Helicobacter pylori*

Helicobacter pylori infection of the gastric epithelium is associated with gastritis, gastric ulcer and duodenal ulcer. Testing for the presence of *H. pylori* in patients with dyspepsia identifies those that may benefit from empirical eradication treatment. Non-invasive tests are:

- Serology (IgG antibody test)—identifies past infection, but is not useful as a test for successful eradication after treatment.
- Urea breath test—can be used to confirm eradication after treatment.
- Stool antigen testing—can be used to confirm eradication 12 weeks or more after eradication therapy.

Invasive tests which can reliably confirm eradication of *H. pylori* after treatment include:

- Mucosal biopsy and histological examination (Gold standard).
- Mucosal biopsy and rapid urease test.

Endoscopy

Endoscopy can be useful to identify:

- Oesophagitis (occurs in 30–40% of patients with GORD).
- Hiatus hernia—this may be noted on endoscopy but itself is not diagnostic of acid reflux because it is often an incidental finding, especially in elderly people.

- Peptic ulcer disease and gastritis—biopsies can be taken to exclude malignancy in gastric ulcers and identify *H. pylori* infection.

Barium meal

This is an alternative for patients for whom endoscopy may be difficult. It may demonstrate ulcer disease or malignancy.

Swallowing problems

Objectives

You should be able to:

- Take a history from a patient with swallowing problems
- Describe the differential diagnosis of dysphagia

DIFFERENTIAL DIAGNOSIS

The patient will usually complain of difficulty swallowing or the sensation of food sticking as it goes down (dysphagia). Difficulty with the passage of food typically begins with solids like bread or meat, followed by liquids if the condition is progressive. The condition is usually painless and is due to a narrowing of the oesophageal lumen.

The differential diagnoses include:

- Oesophageal carcinoma.
- Achalasia.
- Benign oesophageal stricture.
- Oesophagitis.
- Oesophageal spasm.
- Failure of peristalsis due to other reasons (e.g. scleroderma).
- Oesophageal pouch or diverticulum.
- Oesophageal web.
- Incarcerated hiatus hernia.
- Foreign body obstruction.

HISTORY OF THE PATIENT WITH SWALLOWING PROBLEMS

Taking a careful history of the presenting complaint is the key to sorting out the differential diagnosis. Important features to ask about are discussed below.

Duration of symptoms

A long or intermittent history, usually accompanied by manoeuvres to relieve the symptoms, often indicates anatomical or mechanical obstruction due to:

- Pouch.
- Diverticulum.
- Webs.
- Incarcerated hernia.

The first three are more common in younger adults; the last in elderly people.

Level at which dysphagia occurs

Attempt to determine the level at which dysphagia is experienced, as:

- High-level dysphagia can be due to cricopharyngeal spasm, a contraction of the cricopharyngeus muscle and inferior constrictors, which is closely associated with pharyngeal pouch.
- Low-level dysphagia is more common with peptic strictures.
- Carcinoma occurs at all levels (Fig. 2.1)

The patient's perception of the level at which dysphagia occurs is not a reliable indication of the level of obstruction.

Weight loss

Minor weight loss is common because patients may have modified their diet to cope with dysphagia. Significant weight loss is an ominous sign and almost always indicates carcinoma.

History of heartburn

A history of heartburn preceding the dysphagia is highly suggestive of benign oesophageal stricture

Fig. 2.1 Sites at which oesophageal lesions cause dysphagia. The patient will often describe the level of obstruction as high, mid or lower chest but this does not reliably correlate with site or nature of pathology.

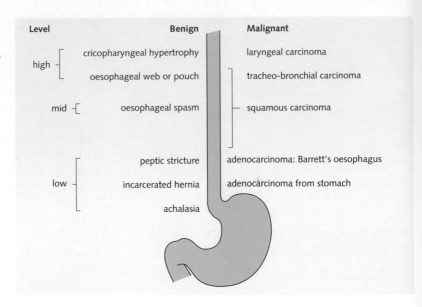

Level	Benign	Malignant
high	cricopharyngeal hypertrophy	laryngeal carcinoma
	oesophageal web or pouch	tracheo-bronchial carcinoma
mid	oesophageal spasm	squamous carcinoma
low	peptic stricture	adenocarcinoma: Barrett's oesophagus
	incarcerated hernia	adenocarcinoma from stomach
	achalasia	

occurring as a result of chronic oesophagitis with subsequent fibrosis. The benign stricture may then reduce further acid reflux leading to a reduced sensation of heartburn.

It is important to ask patients with dysphagia about which types of food produce the worst symptoms. Strictures (including tumours) typically produce dysphagia initially to solids and then, if they progress, to liquids. A combination of dysphagia to both solids and liquids, developing over a few years, may suggest achalasia (a failure of the lower oesophageal sphincter to relax). Chest pain occurs in roughly one-third of patients with achalasia and may get better with time.

Regurgitation of food

- Achalasia: regurgitation may relieve the symptoms of retrosternal discomfort that can occur after food in patients with dysphagia.
- Pharyngeal pouch: incomplete relaxation of the upper oesophageal sphincter can lead to herniation of mucosa through the pharyngeal wall (Zenker's diverticulum). Elderly patients complain of regurgitation and dysphagia and may also have marked halitosis due to retained food residue.

Regurgitation is not a feature of oesophageal carcinoma or benign strictures.

Recurrent pulmonary infections

Dysphagia with or without regurgitation may lead to aspiration and subsequent pulmonary infection.

Progression of dysphagia

Progressive dysphagia is manifest by the patient finding increasing difficulty with soft foods or liquids, following difficulty with solids. This may occur over a relatively short duration (weeks or months) and is an ominous development, most often signifying an oesophageal carcinoma.

Pain with dysphagia

Pain on swallowing is termed odynophagia and may or may not be accompanied by dysphagia. Odynophagia may be caused by:

- Infection with *Candida*—this is the most common cause.
- Herpes and cytomegalovirus (CMV) infection (should trigger investigation for HIV infection).

- Impaction of a foreign body—this may cause dysphagia and will usually have an obvious history (e.g. fish bones represent the most common cause).

Pain between the shoulder blades in association with heartburn usually signifies oesophagitis.

> Oesophageal candidiasis should always prompt the clinician to look for underlying immunosuppression, for example corticosteroids or other immunosuppressive treatments, diabetes, malignancy and advanced HIV disease.

Important past medical history

Find out about the patient's past medical history, particularly:

- Risk factors for carcinoma—these include Barrett's oesophagitis, tylosis (thickening of the palms of the hand and soles of the feet) and smoking.
- Chronic systemic diseases—neuromuscular disorders such as motor neurone disease, myasthenia gravis and myotonia dystrophica are associated with disordered peristalsis.
- Collagen vascular disease, for example scleroderma, which can interfere with the elasticity of the oesophagus and impair peristalsis.

EXAMINING THE PATIENT WITH SWALLOWING PROBLEMS

Look out for:

- Weight loss—if marked, should give cause for concern. Patients with carcinoma are often cachectic. A healthy, well-nourished patient with a history of dysphagia usually indicates a benign aetiology, but not exclusively so.
- Anaemia—sometimes clinically evident, it can occur with oesophagitis and classically has been a feature associated with oesophageal web (Plummer–Vinson or Paterson–Kelly syndrome). It is more common with malignant disease.
- Systemic features—clubbing, tylosis, supraclavicular lymph nodes and hepatomegaly are suggestive of malignant disease in the context of dysphagia.
- An epigastric mass—may be palpable if the tumour extends into the cardia and certainly signifies extensive disease. However, there are no clinical signs that are specific for oesophageal carcinoma.

INVESTIGATING SWALLOWING PROBLEMS

It is imperative to investigate any patient who presents with dysphagia. A summary algorithm is shown in Fig. 2.2.

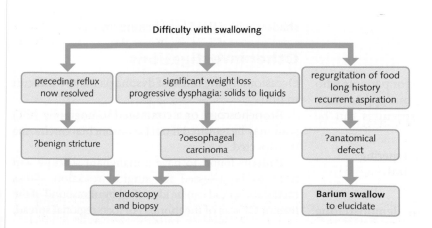

Fig. 2.2 Algorithm for the investigation of a patient with difficulty in swallowing.

11

Acute abdominal pain

Objectives

You should be able to:

- Take a history from a patient with acute abdominal pain
- Understand how to select appropriate investigations for a patient with acute abdominal pain

Acute abdominal pain is a common presentation in clinical medicine and often the most difficult to deal with. It usually refers to pain of sudden onset and a duration of less than 48 hours.

The differential diagnoses of acute abdominal pain include:

- Acute peptic ulceration.
- Biliary colic.
- Acute cholecystitis.
- Acute pancreatitis.
- Acute appendicitis.
- Acute diverticulitis.
- Perforation of abdominal viscus.
- Bowel obstruction.
- Acute renal colic, pyelonephritis or acute urinary retention.
- Acute infarction of bowel, spleen or kidney.
- Myocardial infarction—occasionally presents with acute upper abdominal pain (particularly in the elderly).
- Acute hepatic vein thrombosis (Budd–Chiari syndrome).
- Lower lobe pneumonia—can present with referred abdominal pain.
- Rupture of an abdominal aortic aneurysm.
- Metabolic causes: diabetic ketoacidosis, Addison's disease, acute intermittent porphyria.
- Gynaecological causes: ectopic pregnancy, acute salpingitis, ovarian cyst rupture.

It is important to organize management (e.g. intravenous access, analgesia, etc.) at the same time as attempting to make a diagnosis.

HISTORY OF THE PATIENT WITH ACUTE ABDOMINAL PAIN

A carefully elicited history is vital in helping to discern the cause of acute abdominal pain. The following points should be considered.

Site of pain

The site of pain gives the most important clue to its cause (see Fig. 21.1). Acute epigastric pain is suggestive of:

- Peptic ulcer disease.
- Acute pancreatitis.
- Biliary colic.

By contrast, acute lower abdominal pain is suggestive of:

- Gynaecological problems (e.g. acute salpingitis).
- Acute appendicitis.
- Acute diverticulitis.
- Acute urinary retention.

Particular sites of pain tend to be associated with specific conditions, for example:

- Pain in the right iliac fossa due to appendicitis.
- Pain in the right upper quadrant due to acute cholecystitis.
- Pain in the left iliac fossa due to acute diverticulitis.
- Pain in the loin due to renal colic.

Generalized pain is more likely to be due to a metabolic cause or peritonitis from perforation or infarction.

15

Radiation of pain

Pain due to certain conditions characteristically radiates to particular sites. For example:

- Pancreatic pain radiates 'through' to the middle of the back.
- Gall bladder pain commonly radiates around the right side to the back.
- Myocardial pain, when caused by ischaemia in the diaphragmatic surface, radiates to the epigastrium.
- Renal pain starts in the loin but radiates to the groin.

Character of the pain

The character may be difficult to ascertain and is not always reliable, but the following may be useful:

- 'Colicky' describes pain that builds to a crescendo and subsides. It is characteristic of hollow organ pain (e.g. distension of the bowel, bile duct or ureter wall in obstruction). It implies spasm of the smooth muscle wall of the viscus, often due to obstruction (e.g. ureteric calculus).
- A sharp stabbing pain worsened by movement or respiration suggests pleural or peritoneal irritation (e.g. peritonitis from acute appendicitis or cholecystitis).

Generalized peritonitis has a similar characteristic, but is less well localized and is seen with perforation or ruptured aortic aneurysm.

Relieving and exacerbating factors

These are not often helpful in the acute situation. With any painful condition, the patient will usually adopt the most comfortable posture:

- Peptic ulcer disease may reveal a history of pain exacerbated or relieved by food.
- Acute pancreatitis is classically relieved by sitting forward while holding the abdomen.
- Vomiting may relieve the pain of bowel obstruction.

Past medical history

Past history and risk factors are important, for example:

- In an elderly patient with known abdominal aortic aneurysm, a sudden onset of abdominal pain may be due to rupture.

- A patient with a history of constipation may present with acute obstruction.

Risk factors for acute pancreatitis include:

- Gallstones.
- Alcohol.
- Recent endoscopic retrograde cholangiopancreatography (ERCP).

Family history

This may be relevant (e.g. porphyria is a hereditary condition that commonly presents with acute abdominal pain).

A menstrual history accompanied by a urinary human chorionic gonadotrophin test is essential to exclude the possibility of a ruptured ectopic pregnancy.

EXAMINING THE PATIENT WITH ACUTE ABDOMINAL PAIN

A general inspection can reveal a lot about your patient while you are taking the history and instigating management. Decide whether the patient looks 'ill'. This is a good indicator of serious underlying pathology. Other pointers are:

- Is the patient lying still with shallow breathing (generalized peritonitis)?
- Is the patient agitated and restless (colicky pain) or holding a particular part of the abdomen (localized peritonitis)?
- Is the patient tachycardic, peripherally cool and/or hypotensive, suggesting hypovolaemic shock (ruptured abdominal aneurysm, ectopic pregnancy)?
- Is there any external bruising (acute pancreatitis)?
- Is the patient tachypnoeic (a sign of significant metabolic acidosis)?
- Is there a fever indicative of an infective or inflammatory process?

Guarding and rebound tenderness

If the patient tends to hold the abdominal muscle rigid (guarding), this may suggest peritonitis is present. The abdomen will be tender but the patient will allow gradual gentle pressure. Sudden removal of the palpating hand produces rebound tenderness—this is an important sign of peritonitis which can also be elicited by the patient being reluctant to 'blow out' the abdomen to touch your hand positioned at about 5 cm above the resting abdomen.

Site of tenderness

If tenderness is more localized, think of the underlying structure, for example:

- Appendix in the right iliac fossa.
- Descending colon in the left iliac fossa.
- Ovaries in the lower abdomen.
- Stomach or pancreas in the upper abdomen.

Pulsation

A pulsating or expansile mass may suggest an aortic aneurysm but, in some cases of rupture, the pulsation may be absent. Peripheral pulses should be palpated.

Beware of a ruptured abdominal aortic aneurysm masquerading as a history of renal colic, particularly in older patients with arterial disease.

Distension

Acute obstruction of the small or large bowel can cause painful abdominal distension with a resonant percussion note. In the presence of chronic liver disease, ascites may be present and can become infected (spontaneous bacterial peritonitis, SBP). Acute onset of painful ascites is sometimes seen in hepatic vein thrombosis (Budd–Chiari syndrome).

Hernial orifices and male genitalia

Examination of the hernial orifices (inguinal and femoral) is important to exclude the possibility of an incarcerated hernia giving rise to small bowel obstruction. Testicular torsion can also manifest as lower abdominal pain.

Internal examination

Rectal examination is essential to exclude melaena from acute upper gastrointestinal ulceration. Constipation may give a clue about obstruction or a tender rectal examination may be due to a locally inflamed retrocaecal appendix.

Vaginal examination may be indicated in certain circumstances (e.g. a tender fornix may suggest torsion or rupture of an ovarian cyst).

INVESTIGATING ACUTE ABDOMINAL PAIN

Investigations are usually important to confirm your diagnosis or to determine the severity of the illness.

Full blood count

A full blood count may aid diagnosis:

- A raised white cell count may support a diagnosis of underlying sepsis or peritonitis, but is relatively non-specific. There may be haemoconcentration due to dehydration, manifest by a high/normal haemoglobin and supported by an elevated urea.
- Platelets will be high in inflammatory disease or chronic gastrointestinal blood loss.
- A low haemoglobin should raise suspicion of bleeding in association with the acute abdominal pain.

Biochemistry

Specific biochemical tests and their correct interpretation in the context of acute abdominal pain can be very helpful:

- A raised amylase is important to support a diagnosis of acute pancreatitis, but it can be slightly raised in cholecystitis, biliary colic, ectopic pregnancy, perforated peptic ulcer and other intra-abdominal catastrophes.
- Urea and electrolytes may be disturbed if the patient is ill or dehydrated. The combination

of hyperkalaemia with hyponatraemia should suggest the possibility of Addison's disease.

- A high sugar with acidosis in a patient with acute abdominal pain may be due to diabetic ketoacidosis.
- Abnormal liver enzymes may help make the diagnosis of pain due to gallstone disease with obstructive jaundice or Budd–Chiari syndrome, for example.
- Hypercalcaemia can cause constipation and abdominal pain.
- Urine analysis may reveal haematuria suggestive of renal colic, or nitrites and leucocytes indicative of a urinary tract infection.
- Urinary porphyrin estimation has been superseded by measurement of specific enzyme activity in the blood.
- A pregnancy test is mandatory in women of childbearing age.
- C-reactive protein is a sensitive acute phase protein indicative of ongoing infection or inflammation, and it would be unusual for this to be normal in any significant cause of acute abdominal pain.

A low venous bicarbonate or arterial blood gas analysis consistent with metabolic acidosis is suggestive of acute intra-abdominal pathology (e.g. bowel infarction, pancreatitis or peritonitis).

Radiology

An erect chest radiograph is essential to exclude air under the diaphragm, indicative of a perforated intra-abdominal viscus (Fig. 3.1).

A plain abdominal X-ray may reveal:

- Dilated bowel loops indicative of obstruction (Fig. 3.2).
- Faecal loading associated with constipation or obstruction.
- Calcification in gallstones, ureteric stones (commonly radio-opaque) or aortic aneurysm.

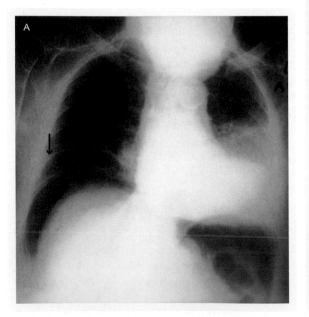
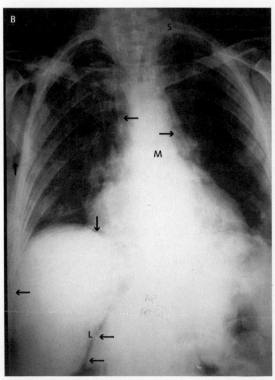

Fig. 3.1 Chest X-rays. (A) A patient with acute abdominal pain due to visceral perforation. Air under the diaphragm is more obvious on the right side above the liver (arrows). (B) A patient with retroperitoneal perforation: arrows show where air tracks up around the liver (L), into the mediastinum (M) and subcutaneously (S) (felt as crackling under the skin).

Ultrasound is not routinely performed as an emergency, but may be helpful in confirming:

- Dilated bile ducts due to stones.
- Stones in the gallbladder.
- Congested liver (Budd–Chiari).
- Ovarian cysts.

Similarly, a computed tomography (CT) scan is rarely needed in the emergency situation, but can be useful when the diagnosis is not apparent (e.g. ruptured liver or renal cysts), or if a ruptured aortic aneurysm is suspected.

Electrocardiography

All patients who present with chest or abdominal pain should have an electrocardiogram to exclude myocardial infarction (Fig. 3.3). Some T-wave changes are non-specific and can be seen in many causes of acute abdominal pain, although ultimately cardiac enzyme levels may need to be measured to exclude myocardial injury.

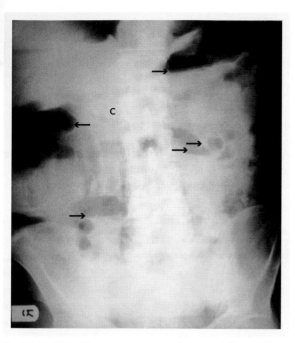

Fig. 3.2 Abdominal X-ray from a patient with intestinal obstruction, showing fluid levels in the bowel (arrows), a grossly distended caecum (C) and a collapsed colon.

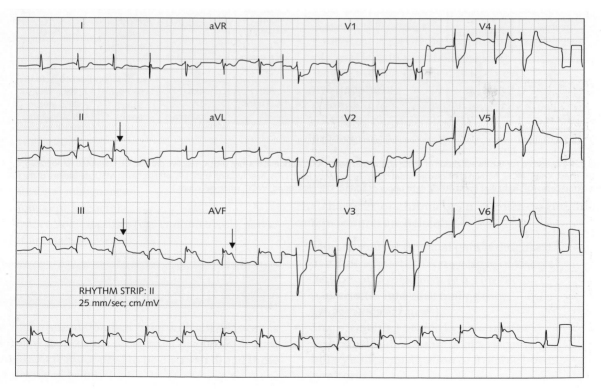

Fig. 3.3 Electrocardiogram from a patient presenting with acute abdominal pain. ST segment elevation in leads II, III and AVF (arrows) supports a diagnosis of inferior myocardial infarction.

Take a history of each episode of pain. Has hospital admission been necessary? Evaluation of old medical notes can be very revealing.

Exacerbating and relieving factors

These are sometimes helpful. The patient may have had the pain for some time and may have experimented with ways to relieve or exacerbate the pain, such as with food or alcohol.

Food can have the following effects:

- It may aggravate biliary causes, characteristically occurring 20–30 minutes after a meal, and there may be fat intolerance, although this is not specific for a particular diagnosis.
- With mesenteric ischaemia ('abdominal angina'), patients may notice that pain occurs 1–2 hours after food and this results in a reluctance to eat, for fear of pain.
- It can relieve the pain of a duodenal ulcer, particularly if the patient drinks milk at bedtime.

Alcohol:

- Worsens chronic pancreatitis and gastritis, but the patient does not always modify his or her behaviour.

Defaecation or passage of flatus:

- Relieves lower abdominal pain due to constipation or irritable bowel.
- May exacerbate pain due to local inflammatory conditions of the anus or rectum, or in obstruction.

Menstruation:

- Painful periods should be obvious but ectopic areas of endometriosis may also induce pain at the time of menstruation.
- Pain in mid cycle can occur with ovulation ('mittelschmerz') or occasionally with ovarian cysts.

Associated features

Patients may not notice other symptoms or realize their significance in relation to the pain. It is therefore important to ask specifically about:

- Distension or bloating—if intermittent, this is suggestive of irritable bowel syndrome or subacute obstruction; if progressive, it may indicate development of a mass or ascites.
- Weight loss—think of underlying malignancy (i.e. pancreatic or intestinal), especially in elderly patients. In younger patients, think of Crohn's disease or lymphoma. Weight loss may also result from avoidance of food.
- Change in bowel habit—alternating constipation or diarrhoea may be due to a change in diet but intestinal malignancy must be excluded in patients aged over 45 years.
- Rectal bleeding—may signify an underlying inflammatory or malignant process (see Ch. 10).
- Vaginal discharge—pelvic inflammatory disease is something the patient may be embarrassed to volunteer information about.

Many patients will be reluctant to reveal their level of alcohol consumption. Careful questioning is often required! Try to ascertain their habit from several angles.

EXAMINING THE PATIENT WITH CHRONIC ABDOMINAL PAIN

On general inspection, important features to note include:

- Obvious signs of weight loss.
- Pigmentation, pallor or jaundice.
- Signs of dehydration.

In the neck, look for:

- Lymphadenopathy, particularly in the supraclavicular regions.
- Goitre.

Abdominal inspection and palpation may reveal:

- Scars from previous surgery—patients occasionally omit information about previous operations.
- Distension—is it uniform due to ascites or asymmetrical due to a mass?
- Peristalsis may be obvious in thin people with intestinal obstruction.

- A mass may be present, and its anatomical location usually indicates the aetiology (e.g. epigastric in gastric malignancy, right iliac fossa in Crohn's disease, or an appendix mass).
- Stigmata of chronic alcohol misuse may be present (spider naevi, umbilical varices and other signs of chronic liver disease).

Other features to note are:

- Signs of peripheral vascular disease which may accompany mesenteric ischaemia.
- Tenderness in the fornix or vaginal discharge, suggesting pelvic inflammatory disease.
- Rectal examination should always be performed for patients with lower abdominal pain.

INVESTIGATING CHRONIC ABDOMINAL PAIN

Full blood count

Anaemia may be due to blood loss giving rise to a microcytic hypochromic picture of iron deficiency. In malignant or inflammatory disease, a normocytic anaemia may also occur. Raised white cell count is indicative of underlying infection or inflammation. Platelets can be raised in chronic inflammatory disease or chronic gastrointestinal blood loss.

> Iron deficiency anaemia in the context of chronic abdominal pain should always prompt endoscopic examination of either the upper or lower gastrointestinal tract (or both—in context with the clinical findings).

Biochemistry

Often a range of biochemistry tests is undertaken as a routine, but it is essential to interpret these in the clinical context. The following may be helpful:

- Electrolytes can be disturbed if diarrhoea or vomiting have occurred (e.g. low potassium).
- Calcium can be raised in malignant disease, but hypercalcaemia for other reasons (e.g. hyperparathyroidism) may also cause chronic abdominal pain.

- Amylase can be raised slightly and non-specifically with many causes of abdominal pain. It is usually normal in chronic pancreatitis, in contradistinction to acute pancreatitis.
- Liver enzyme abnormalities are common with cholangitis or gallstone problems.
- Urea may be raised if dehydration is present, or low if the patient has been anorectic, has malabsorption or has liver disease.
- A thyroid function test should be performed because hypothyroidism is an occasional cause of abdominal pain.

Radiology

Although often unrevealing, a plain abdominal radiograph may reveal:

- Calcification indicative of chronic pancreatitis (Fig. 4.1). Ten per cent of gallstones are radio-opaque.
- Faecal loading suggestive of chronic constipation.
- Dilated bowel indicative of subacute obstruction.

Abdominal ultrasound is useful to identify:

- Gallstones causing chronic cholecystitis or bile duct obstruction.
- Liver metastases which commonly arise from the colon or breast (Fig. 4.2).
- Chronic pancreatitis or carcinoma of the body of the pancreas.
- Intra-abdominal lymphadenopathy—suggesting lymphoma or metastatic disease.

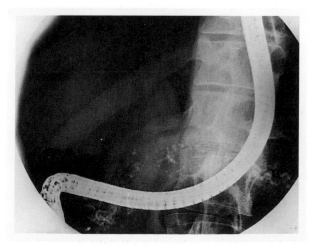

Fig. 4.1 Abdominal calcification is seen across the pancreatic area in a pre-injection endoscopic retrograde cholangiopancreatogram.

Fig. 4.2 Ultrasound scan showing multiple areas of different echogenicity and size in the liver suggestive of metastases.

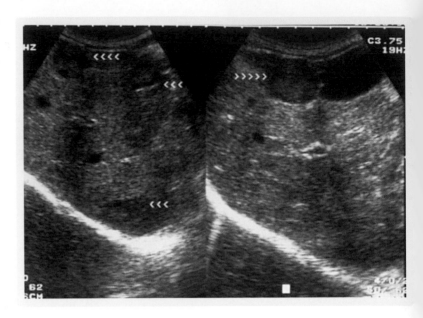

Contrast studies can be helpful:

- Small bowel barium enema can be used to identify stricture in the terminal ileum due to Crohn's disease.
- Large bowel barium enema is used to confirm diverticular disease or exclude colonic carcinoma.

Computed tomography of the abdomen may be required to visualize chronic pancreatitis or pancreatic carcinoma and to search for, or stage, lymphoma.

Endoscopy

Gastroscopy is useful to investigate dyspepsia (see Ch. 1) and to exclude gastric carcinoma. Colonoscopy may be required to confirm diverticular disease or to exclude colonic carcinoma.

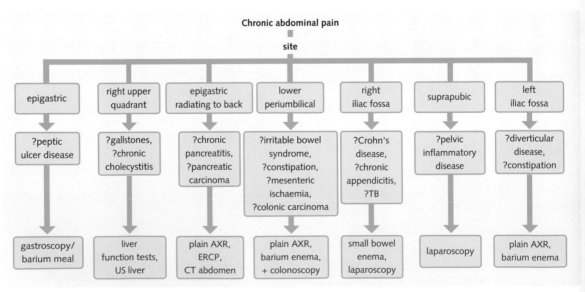

Fig. 4.3 Algorithm for the investigation of chronic abdominal pain. (AXR, abdominal X-ray; CT, computed tomography; ERCP, endoscopic retrograde cholangiopancreatography; US, ultrasound.)

Surgery

Despite extensive (and sometimes expensive!) investigation, no cause for chronic abdominal pain may be found. In this situation, and after careful consideration, a diagnostic laparoscopy can be useful (e.g. to identify endometriosis).

Summary

An algorithm summarizing the investigation of chronic abdominal pain is shown in Fig. 4.3.

Abdominal distension 5

Objectives

You should be able to:

- Take a history from a patient with abdominal distension
- List the causes of ascites

Swelling of the abdomen rarely presents in isolation: it usually accompanies other symptoms such as abdominal pain, diarrhoea, jaundice or weight loss.

HISTORY OF THE PATIENT WITH ABDOMINAL DISTENSION

Patients may complain that their abdomen is abnormally distended. They may have noticed that their clothes are fitting too tightly. Others may have commented that they have put on weight or look pregnant.

Occasionally, patients do not realize they have abdominal distension until it is detected on physical examination. Several specific features in the history can give important clues to the aetiology or pathogenesis.

Traditionally, all medical students are taught abdominal distension is caused by Fat, Faeces, Flatus, Fluid or Fetus (the five Fs) and, although this is not strictly accurate, it is worth remembering, especially when one comes across a difficult examiner!

Onset of symptoms

The onset may give a clue about its cause:

- Distension caused by ascites often takes several days or weeks to develop and progresses with time (Fig. 5.1).

- Acute abdominal distension accompanied by pain suggests the diagnosis of Budd–Chiari syndrome (i.e. hepatic vein thrombosis).
- Distension due to acute bowel obstruction may only have a relatively short period of onset (i.e. 12–24 hours) and will have associated features such as vomiting, abdominal pain and absolute constipation. The more proximal the site of obstruction, the less marked will be the abdominal distension.
- Menstrual history is important in women of childbearing age: unexpected pregnancies occur and have occasionally gone unnoticed or been denied, even up to full term.
- Intermittent distension is suggestive of subacute obstruction or, more commonly, irritable bowel syndrome, in which patients obtain relief from opening their bowels.

Causes of ascites	
High protein (exudative)	**Low protein (transudative) >10 g^{+-} less than serum albumin**
- intra-abdominal malignancy (primary or secondary) - infection (especially TB) - pancreatitis - Budd–Chiari syndrome	- hypoalbuminaemia (from any cause, e.g. nephrotic syndrome) - cirrhosis - cardiac failure or constrictive pericarditis

Fig. 5.1 Causes of ascites—differentiated by protein concentration of ascitic fluid. Protein level should be compared to serum albumin concentration, and correlated with cell count, culture, cytology and amylase level in fluid.

Bowel habit

Abdominal distension due to gastrointestinal disease will usually be associated with a disturbance of gastrointestinal function.

A long history of constipation may suggest that the distension is due to faeces. In severe cases, subacute or acute obstruction occurs and the distension is further aggravated by flatus. Abdominal pain and vomiting may also be a prominent feature.

Alternating diarrhoea and constipation associated with intermittent distension and borborygmi are highly suggestive of irritable bowel syndrome.

Past history

As always, the patient's past medical history can give helpful clues:

- A history of liver disease may suggest ascites.
- Pericardial disease due to rheumatic fever in the past, or even tuberculosis, can produce constrictive pericarditis, and is often forgotten as a cause of ascites.
- Cardiac failure can also cause ascites.
- Nephrotic syndrome can result in hypoalbuminaemic ascites.

A family history may be important (e.g. polycystic kidney or polycystic liver disease, which can produce distension if cysts are large). The condition is autosomal dominant.

EXAMINING THE PATIENT WITH ABDOMINAL DISTENSION

On general examination, several features can be helpful:

- Presence of jaundice, parotitis or encephalo-pathy suggests the possibility of liver-related ascites.
- The patient may not be able to lie down flat for the examination due to pulmonary oedema, secondary to congestive cardiac failure.
- Truncal obesity together with abdominal striae may alert one to the diagnosis of Cushing's disease.

- A paradoxical rise in the jugular venous pulse on inspiration may suggest constrictive pericarditis, and the heart sounds may be diminished.

On examination of the abdomen:

- Look for any asymmetry present—is the lower abdomen more distended? This may be the case in pregnancy, urinary retention, ovarian tumour or fibroids protruding from the pelvic cavity (Fig. 5.2).
- Look for scars that may be present—has the patient had previous surgery for malignancy or obstruction?
- Faecal loading is often palpable over the descending colon and can be indented, unlike a malignant mass.
- Hepatosplenomegaly may be evident if underlying cirrhosis or right ventricular failure is present.
- A rectal examination is mandatory for masses arising from the pelvis.
- Supplemental vaginal examination may be required if an ovarian or uterine origin is suspected.

Percussion of the abdomen is most helpful in differentiating types of distension:

- A tympanic note is produced by gaseous distension.
- A dull note is produced by a solid mass.
- 'Shifting dullness' is demonstrable when a dull note in the flank becomes resonant following the patient rolling onto the opposite side. This suggests gravity-dependent free fluid in the abdomen (i.e. ascites).

Auscultation can be useful in complete obstruction, when bowel sounds may be hyperactive (often described as tinkling) or absent.

INVESTIGATING ABDOMINAL DISTENSION

Investigation is largely influenced by the clinical scenario, but radiological investigation has a key role in differentiating between causes of abdominal distension.

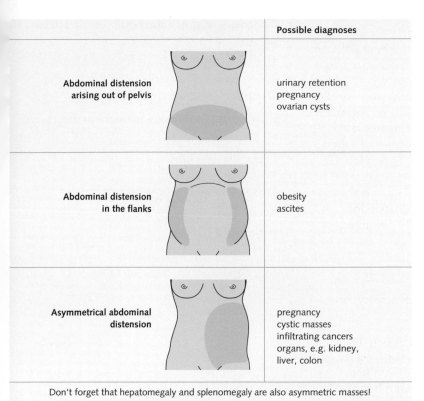

Fig. 5.2 Illustration of patterns of abdominal distension.

	Possible diagnoses
Abdominal distension arising out of pelvis	urinary retention pregnancy ovarian cysts
Abdominal distension in the flanks	obesity ascites
Asymmetrical abdominal distension	pregnancy cystic masses infiltrating cancers organs, e.g. kidney, liver, colon

Don't forget that hepatomegaly and splenomegaly are also asymmetric masses!

Radiology

Different imaging modalities may be used for diagnosis:

- Chest X-ray is useful to demonstrate an enlarged heart or signs of cardiac failure. In constrictive pericarditis, the heart border may appear calcified and heart size may be normal.
- Plain abdominal X-ray is indicated if the patient is suspected clinically of having bowel obstruction. This can be seen as dilated loops of bowel. An erect abdominal X-ray may show fluid levels (see Fig. 3.2). Occasionally, a calcified mass may be seen in the pelvis due to fibroids or dermoid cysts of the ovaries. Faecal loading may also be shown in the colon.
- Abdominal ultrasound is the diagnostic modality of choice to identify ascites. It is also helpful to differentiate pelvic from intra-abdominal masses.
- A computed tomography or magnetic resonance imaging scan of the abdomen may be indicated

for some patients when ultrasound is equivocal (Fig. 5.3) or for a diagnosis of underlying malignancy.

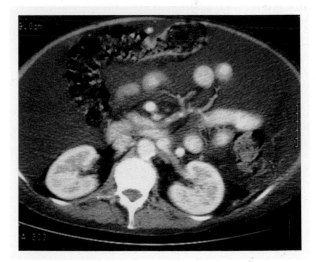

Fig. 5.3 Distension caused by ascites (ground glass appearance). Small bowel is floating in the fluid.

A pregnancy test is essential if the cause of abdominal distension is not obvious for other reasons in women of childbearing age. This is achieved by measuring the level of human chorionic gonadotrophin in the urine. Protein in the urine should alert one to the possibility of nephrotic syndrome.

Electrocardiogram may show:

- Elevated ST segment.
- T-wave changes.
- Low voltage QRS complexes (if a pericardial effusion is present).

Echocardiography is useful to demonstrate:

- Valvular stenosis or regurgitation.
- Pericardial effusion.
- Pericardial thickening.
- Poor ventricular myocardial function.

Cardiac investigation

Further tests may be necessary if cardiac failure or constrictive pericarditis is considered likely.

Summary

An algorithm summarizing the investigation of abdominal distension is shown in Fig. 5.4.

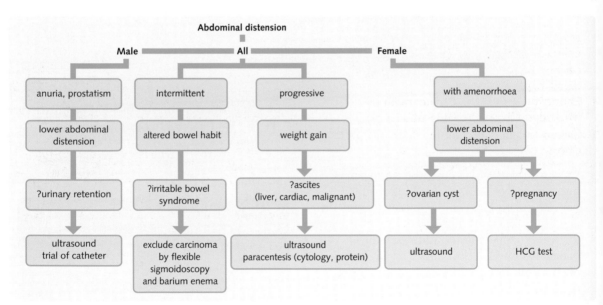

Fig. 5.4 Algorithm for the investigation of abdominal distension. (HCG, human chorionic gonadotrophin.)

Weight loss and anorexia

Weight loss can be a very subjective assessment and, for a comprehensive investigation, it is important to try to attain objective evidence so that the rate and quantity of weight loss can be ascertained. Anorexia is loss of appetite which commonly accompanies weight loss, and it is appropriate to consider these entities together.

The causes are myriad and include:

- Malignancy of any variety due to hypermetabolic effects. Gastrointestinal (GI) malignancy clearly can also cause weight loss by interfering with the digestive process.
- Endocrine causes (e.g. diabetes mellitus, hyperthyroidism, adrenal insufficiency).
- Malabsorption (e.g. coeliac disease, Crohn's disease, bacterial overgrowth, intestinal parasitosis, chronic pancreatitis).
- Infection (e.g. underlying abscess, tuberculosis).
- Psychiatric cause (e.g. anorexia nervosa or bulimia, depression).
- Neurological cause (e.g. bulbar palsy, myasthenia causing difficulty in swallowing).

Documentation of weight over a period of time is often extremely useful (e.g. clinic notes, general practitioner records). For reasons of posterity, it is important to document weight at every opportunity when you clerk a patient.

HISTORY OF THE PATIENT WITH WEIGHT LOSS

An inquisitive history is required to assess weight loss objectively. Important aspects to enquire about include:

- How much weight loss and over what period of time? Weight loss of 10 kg over 2 months is clearly more significant than over 1 year.
- Do their clothes fit them more loosely? How much tighter do belts have to be?
- Do they have any recent photographs to compare weight over a period of time?

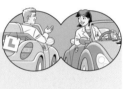

Some personality traits occur often in patients with anorexia nervosa. Careful questioning about life at home and school can be very revealing. Young females with anorexia often have a desire for perfection and perform well academically. They tend to be socially isolated. Up to 50% of patients with anorexia nervosa have depression and, in fact, suicide is a more common cause of death in these patients than starvation.

Anorexia

It is very important to assess appetite when considering weight loss. The following should be considered:

- Are there any features of psychiatric illness such as distorted body image, early wakening, depression, behavioural changes?
- Is appetite out of step with weight loss? Hyperthyroidism causes increased appetite with weight loss. Brain tumours occasionally present with 'omniphagia'.

Associated features

These may give a clue to underlying disease, especially those resulting in malabsorption. Look for any GI symptoms such as:

- Diarrhoea or steatorrhoea (malabsorption, inflammatory bowel disease, hyperthyroidism).
- Vomiting.
- Change in bowel habit (possible malignancy).
- Increased activity due to change of lifestyle.
- Excessive thirst (polydipsia) or excessive passage of urine (polyuria) suggestive of diabetes mellitus.
- Fever, heat intolerance or night sweats, suggesting underlying infection or malignancy.

Although amenorrhoea is characteristic of anorexia nervosa, it will occur with any condition causing profound weight loss. It should also be differentiated from primary amenorrhoea or pituitary failure.

Past medical history

A history of previous GI surgery, particularly partial gastrectomy or small bowel resection, is important, because this may interfere with normal digestion. Patients who have had a stroke or neuromuscular problem such as myasthenia may find chewing or swallowing difficult.

EXAMINING THE PATIENT WITH WEIGHT LOSS

There may be obvious cachexia or weight loss when looking at the patient. Look out for additional signs such as:

- Pallor indicative of anaemia, which may accompany malabsorption, malignancy or chronic infection/inflammation.
- Lymphadenopathy, suggestive of malignancy or lymphoma.
- Tremor with exophthalmos and a goitre, suggestive of thyrotoxicosis.
- Pigmentation of the skin and buccal membrane with postural hypotension, suggesting adrenal insufficiency.

- Hepatomegaly, ascites or jaundice, suggesting possible malignancy or liver abscess.
- Lack of eye contact, withdrawn demeanour or unkempt appearance, suggestive of depression or self-neglect.

Abdominal and particularly rectal examination must not be omitted when considering weight loss.

In a young female who is very thin, the following features ought to arouse suspicion of anorexia nervosa or bulimia:

- A history of excessive dieting or of binge eating.
- Delayed sexual maturation or amenorrhoea.
- Tooth erosion (due to acidic vomiting).
- Wearing loose clothes to disguise a perceived distorted body image.
- Lanugo hair on the arms and trunk.
- Callosities on dorsum of fingers from repeated self-induction of gag-reflex vomiting.

Weight loss in an elderly patient may be due to many factors, and unnecessary, invasive investigations may be avoided in some patients. Chronic disease and increasing frailty can result in reduced appetite and poor nutrition. Depression is common in the elderly and may manifest as loss of interest in food and weight loss. It is important to ask about a patient's home circumstances and family members may have insight into a recent cognitive decline. Are they coping at home? Who cooks?

INVESTIGATING WEIGHT LOSS

A broad spectrum of investigations may be necessary to establish the aetiology of weight loss. The following investigations are confined to weight loss of GI causes and those that may present to a gastroenterologist.

A careful drug history is important. Enquire about laxative abuse and recreational drugs such as amphetamines—both of which can lead to weight loss.

Blood tests

The following blood tests may aid diagnosis:

- A full blood count is important to look for anaemia. A pancytopaenia may be indicative of marrow failure (e.g. malignant infiltration) or malabsorption of vitamin B_{12} or folate, resulting in megaloblastic change.
- Erythrocyte sedimentation rate is a useful test in this context because it is almost always raised if significant malignant or infectious pathology is present. C-reactive protein is a more sensitive marker of inflammatory disease.
- A coagulopathy and low blood urea are indicative of profound malabsorption or malnutrition.
- Measurement of blood sugar is essential to exclude diabetes mellitus.
- Hyperkalaemia with hyponatraemia should arouse suspicion of adrenal insufficiency. A Synacthen test may be indicated.
- Raised liver enzymes in the absence of discernible liver problems should arouse suspicion of malignant disease.
- Thyroid function tests are essential to exclude hyperthyroidism.
- Gonadal function tests may be useful to differentiate primary and secondary causes of amenorrhoea.

- Tumour markers can occasionally be helpful if other investigations prove unrevealing, but need to be interpreted with caution (see Ch. 24).

Radiology

The tests that will be most helpful depend on the clinical context:

- Chest radiograph: exclude occult lung tumour (especially in a smoker), lymphadenopathy (lymphoma), tuberculosis.
- Ultrasound of the abdomen and pelvis is useful to look for underlying malignancy.
- Barium enema should be performed in older age groups to exclude colonic malignancy. In younger patients, a small bowel enema may be indicated to look for evidence of Crohn's disease.
- Computed tomography of the abdomen is the best modality to look for occult malignancy such as pancreatic tumours and intra-abdominal lymphadenopathy.

Endoscopy

Gastroscopy:

- May be important to exclude occult gastric carcinoma in elderly patients.

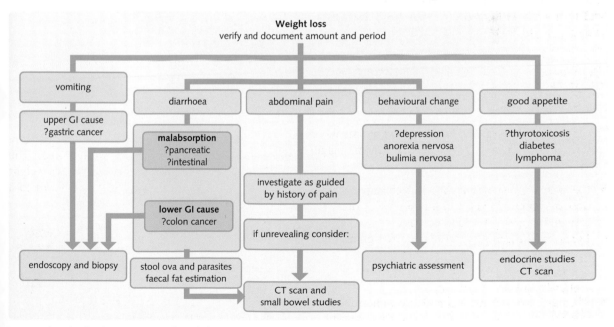

Fig. 6.1 Algorithm for the investigation of weight loss. (CT, computed tomography.)

- Is a useful investigation in younger patients allowing a small bowel biopsy to be taken to exclude coeliac disease.

Colonoscopy may be necessary to evaluate further any lesion in the colon found on barium enema.

Summary

An algorithm summarizing the investigation of weight loss is shown in Fig. 6.1.

Vomiting

Objectives

You should be able to:

- Take a history from a patient with vomiting
- Describe features in a history that help discriminate between gastrointestinal, metabolic and psychogenic causes of vomiting

Vomiting is the forceful ejection of gastric contents through the mouth. It is most often mediated through a vagal reflex involving chemoreceptor trigger zones in the medulla of the brain. It can be differentiated from regurgitation of oesophageal contents due to obstruction or pouch because of its greater force and volume. It is frequently preceded by nausea or abdominal pain. Vomiting can also occur because of intracranial phenomena or direct toxic effects on the trigger zone by drugs.

The common causes of vomiting include:

- Drug toxicity.
- Vestibular disturbances.
- Gastric causes such as gastritis, consequent upon alcohol excess, noxious substances, viral infection, bile, non-steroidal anti-inflammatory drugs.
- Pregnancy.
- Migraine.
- Liver disease such as acute hepatitis or hepatic failure.
- Gastrointestinal (GI) obstruction due to malignancy/pyloric stenosis/herniae/adhesions/ volvulus/stricture.
- Gastroparesis secondary to autonomic dysfunction (e.g. diabetes mellitus).
- Metabolic derangement (e.g. adrenal insufficiency, uraemia, hypercalcaemia, porphyria, diabetic ketoacidosis).
- Raised intracranial pressure or inflammation of the brain lining: meningitis or encephalitis.
- Psychogenic vomiting.

HISTORY AND DIFFERENTIAL DIAGNOSIS OF VOMITING

A detailed history is important to differentiate GI from central nervous systems (CNS) causes. Psychogenic or metabolic causes can be very difficult to discern, but are often more chronic or recurrent than is the case with GI causes. Features to consider are discussed below.

Onset and duration

Onset is an important feature: a short history is more likely to be due to an acute cause similar to those seen in acute abdominal pain (e.g. infection or acute intestinal obstruction).

A diagnosis that can be easily missed as a cause of vomiting is a brain neoplasm. Frontal lobe tumours can become quite large before neurological signs are evident. Patients with unexplained, persistent vomiting should have a careful neurological examination and a low threshold for brain imaging.

Drugs and alcohol

A drug history is essential: probably the most common cause of nausea and vomiting.

The list of drugs causing nausea or vomiting is exhaustive, but particular ones to note are:

- Opiates, from codeine to diamorphine.
- Cytotoxic drugs.
- Antibiotics (e.g. erythromycin).
- Digoxin toxicity.

Alcohol excess results in gastritis, and vomiting commonly occurs the morning after excessive alcohol intake.

Infections and toxins

Gastroenteritis (infection in the gastrointestinal tract) is usually of rapid onset and is self-limiting. It manifests as vomiting, abdominal pain and diarrhoea. Older people are commonly affected.

The highly infectious noroviruses (formerly called Norwalk viruses after the school in Norwalk, Ohio where the original outbreak occurred) are the commonest cause of non-bacterial gastroenteritis. Noroviruses are commonly responsible for outbreaks in hospitals, nursing homes and schools. They have become known as the 'cruise ship virus' after well-publicized outbreaks on cruise liners. Symptoms are usually self-limiting.

Food poisoning is caused by ingestion of bacteria or their toxins in contaminated food (Fig. 7.1).

Past history

In addition to medication the patient may be taking for an unrelated condition, the following may also be of significance:

- Previous gastric surgery may give rise to biliary gastritis causing vomiting.

- Chronic duodenal ulceration can cause pyloric stenosis with gastric outlet obstruction.
- Chronic liver disease progressing to hepatic failure can also cause vomiting.
- Long-standing diabetes can result in gastroparesis and obstruction due to autonomic neuropathy.

Associated features

These can often give a clue to the underlying abnormality:

- Diarrhoea is common with vomiting induced by food poisoning.
- Weight loss may be prominent if underlying malignancy is present.
- Postural hypotension may be apparent if adrenal insufficiency is the cause.
- Headache is usually prominent with any CNS cause.
- Psychological factors, particularly in young females, may have a role in recurrent vomiting without anorexia nervosa.

EXAMINING THE PATIENT WITH VOMITING PROBLEMS

General examination is important to ascertain whether a systemic condition is responsible for the vomiting. Important points to consider are:

- Altered level of consciousness, suggestive of drug toxicity or intracranial pathology.
- Neck stiffness or photophobia, indicative of meningitis.

Fig. 7.1 Bacteria and toxins causing food poisoning

Organism	Food at risk	Incubation (h)	Duration
Bacillus cereus[a]	Reheated or fried rice	1–16	12–24 h
Staphylococcus aureus[a]	Cream, unrefrigerated meat	1–6	6–36 h
Clostridium perfringens[a]	Beef, turkey, chicken	12–24	6–36 h
Vibrio parahaemolyiticus[a]	Shellfish	12–18	2–10 days
Salmonella spp	Eggs, poultry	12–24	1–8 days
Campylobacter jejuni	Milk, chicken, beef	24–240	2–30 days

[a] Toxin-mediated gastroenteritis

- Cachexia which may suggest underlying malignancy.
- Pallor or pigmentation indicating anaemia, hypoadrenalism or renal failure.
- Dehydration which may indicate that vomiting has been severe and prolonged.
- Pyrexia or tachycardia, possibly indicative of sepsis.

Abdominal examination is necessary to establish whether there is any evidence of intestinal obstruction and to identify any masses that may be responsible.

A succussion splash may be present with gastric outlet obstruction.

INVESTIGATING VOMITING PROBLEMS

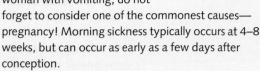

Prior to embarking on a series of investigations in a young woman with vomiting, do not forget to consider one of the commonest causes—pregnancy! Morning sickness typically occurs at 4–8 weeks, but can occur as early as a few days after conception.

Blood tests

Consider the following blood tests:

- Full blood count may support an impression of dehydration if haematocrit is high. Raised white cell count can indicate infection.

- Blood urea is mildly raised in dehydration, but higher levels may be indicative of renal failure or upper GI bleeding which can both cause vomiting.
- Blood glucose is high in diabetic ketoacidosis.
- Hyperkalaemia with hyponatraemia may suggest adrenal insufficiency. Persistent vomiting will also cause hypokalaemic alkalosis (low potassium with elevated bicarbonate).
- Hypercalcaemia from any cause can present with vomiting.
- Liver enzymes may reveal a pattern of acute hepatitis which sometimes presents with vomiting.
- Drug levels (e.g. digoxin) can be useful if drug toxicity is suspected.

Microbiological tests

Blood cultures and cerebrospinal fluid tap may be indicated if the patient is very ill or if meningitis is suspected.

Radiology

Plain abdominal X-ray is useful to exclude obstruction. A computed tomography scan of the head may be indicated by the clinical picture.

Summary

An algorithm summarizing the investigation of vomiting is shown in Fig. 7.2.

radiation colitis, certain bacterial infections and pseudomembranous colitis. Colonic carcinoma can also give rise to blood-stained diarrhoea. Acute gastroenteritis with bloody diarrhoea is associated with infection with *Campylobacter* spp, *Shigella* spp or *Escherichia coli*.

Pale, greasy diarrhoea due to a high fat content (steatorrhoea) is highly indicative of malabsorption, consequent upon small bowel disease or pancreatic insufficiency.

Ask the patient whether:

- There is a history of coeliac disease in the family.
- He or she has consumed excessive alcohol in the past.

There may be associated features that give some clue to the underlying diagnosis, such as:

- Joint pains, mouth ulcers, skin changes or uveitis in inflammatory bowel disease.
- Diabetes mellitus with evidence of peripheral neuropathy in autonomic bowel neuropathy.
- Scleroderma causing hypomotility with malabsorption.
- Jaundice with steatorrhoea due to pancreatitis or pancreatic carcinoma.

Diet

Has the patient's diet changed in any way recently?:

- Increased ingestion of dairy produce.
- High-fibre cereals.
- Stimulants such as coffee.
- Increase in alcohol consumption.

It is surprising how often many patients fail to link intake to output!

Drug history

Diarrhoea commonly occurs with certain drugs:

- Metformin.
- Colchicine.
- Digoxin.
- Purgatives.

Broad-spectrum antibiotics such as the cephalosporins, the penicillins and macrolides (e.g. erythromycin) commonly cause diarrhoea as a result of alteration in gut flora and, in severe cases, pseudomembranous colitis occurs as a result of *Clostridium difficile* overgrowth.

Past medical and surgical history

Find out about:

- Previous vagotomy (e.g. at surgery for peptic ulcer disease) which can result in diarrhoea in some patients.
- Gastric or intestinal surgical resection which can interfere with motility and absorption (e.g. bile salt malabsorption after terminal ileal resection for Crohn's disease).
- Radiotherapy to the abdomen or pelvis for non-gastrointestinal malignancy, such as lymphoma, which may not manifest its adverse gastrointestinal effects until many years later.
- Systemic conditions such as diabetes or collagen-vascular disease which may also cause diarrhoea.
- HIV—predisposes to atypical infections causing diarrhoea such as *Cryptosporidium* (fungal) and cytomegalovirus.

EXAMINING THE PATIENT WITH DIARRHOEA

General features to look for:

- Dehydration is common in acute onset diarrhoea because gastroenteritis is usually associated with vomiting and hence a substantial fluid loss. Large amounts of electrolyte-rich fluid can also be lost in severe diarrhoea seen in inflammatory bowel disease and VIPomas (tumours that secrete vasoactive intestinal peptide).
- Pallor due to anaemia may be seen in inflammatory bowel disease and colonic malignancy due to chronic blood loss, or reflecting the anaemia of chronic disease. Malabsorption can also result in anaemia due to deficiency of iron and vitamin B_{12} or folate.
- Weight loss associated with chronic diarrhoea is a common feature of malabsorption from all causes. Underlying malignancy should also be excluded.
- Associated features of inflammatory bowel disease may be apparent, such as aphthous mouth ulcers, pyoderma gangrenosum and uveitis.
- Associated features of endocrine disease include skin pigmentation in adrenal insufficiency, proptosis or exophthalmos in thyrotoxicosis and peripheral neuropathy in diabetes.

- Clinical features of alcoholic liver disease or of cystic fibrosis may suggest pancreatic insufficiency.
- Look for scars from previous abdominal surgery (see Fig. 22.10).
- Radiotherapy may sometimes produce persistent skin colour changes that are visible for years after treatment. This may be a clue that suggests radiation enteritis.

Patients may forget or omit to tell you that they have had previous intra-abdominal surgery. Remember to examine carefully for scars! Old surgical notes are sometimes valuable, for example:
- Gastric surgery (vagotomy, gastrectomy) can produce diarrhoea
- Pancreatectomy results in malabsorption
- Cholecystectomy or right hemicolectomy can result in bile salt diarrhoea

Palpate for abdominal masses or tenderness. Most gastroenteritis will have associated abdominal discomfort. The finding of a mass in the right iliac fossa may suggest Crohn's disease or a caecal carcinoma.

Rectal examination must be carried out in all patients presenting with diarrhoea.

- Faecal impaction can cause overflow diarrhoea and is common in the elderly.
- A rectal carcinoma may be palpated.

INVESTIGATING DIARRHOEA

The extent of investigation is guided by the severity of diarrhoea and by the information gleaned from the history and examination. As always, correct interpretation of results in the clinical context is most important.

Haematology

Haematology tests may aid diagnosis:

- Full blood count may demonstrate a microcytic hypochromic picture of iron deficiency or macrocytic anaemia resultant upon vitamin B_{12} or folate deficiency (a combined deficiency can produce a normocytic anaemia).
- Microcytic anaemia with altered bowel habit prompts investigation for colon cancer.
- Steatorrhoea with iron deficiency may suggest coeliac disease.

Biochemistry

Consider the following tests:

- Electrolytes may be disrupted if diarrhoea has been severe and prolonged or is caused by adrenal insufficiency.
- Urea is low if malabsorption or malnutrition is present. It is mildly raised in dehydration or in the presence of melaena.
- Iron studies, ferritin, vitamin B_{12} and folate levels may help to interpret associated anaemia (for anaemia, see Ch. 11).
- Thyroid function tests should be performed for any patients who do not clearly have a gastrointestinal cause for the diarrhoea.
- Urinary 5-hydroxyindole acetic acid (5HIAA) is a metabolite of serotonin, which is elevated in carcinoid syndrome (see p. 98).
- Abnormal liver biochemistry may be associated with pancreatic insufficiency, particularly if secondary to chronic alcohol excess.
- A raised C-reactive protein will occur in infective diarrhoea and in active inflammatory bowel disease.

Microbiology

Stool culture is necessary to exclude an underlying infective cause. However, since most infective causes are viral and self-limiting, viral cultures are only carried out in particular circumstances, such as in the immunosuppressed patient. Stool microscopy can be performed to look for ova and cysts seen in parasitic infections such as *Giardia*.

Hospitalized patients, nursing home patients and outpatients who have recently had antibiotics should have stool tested for *Clostridium difficile* toxin.

Radiology

Plain abdominal radiograph can be undertaken:

- To confirm faecal impaction.
- More commonly, to see whether there is a megacolon associated with inflammatory

peri-anal area. Anal tags suggest previously thrombosed haemorrhoids.

- Mucus discharge may be seen in inflammatory bowel disease and anorectal carcinoma.
- Increased anal tone and pain on rectal examination are highly indicative of anal fissure.
- Hard faeces in the rectum may suggest chronic constipation or anal fissure.
- Masses due to rectal carcinoma or polyp can also be palpated on rectal examination.

Proctoscopy enables examination of the position of haemorrhoids, which may be treated with sclerotherapy. Anal fissures can also be seen, although it is unlikely that the patient with this painful condition will tolerate the passage of a proctoscope.

Rigid sigmoidoscopy can visualize up to 15–20 cm from the anal margin, and biopsies can be taken of any suspicious lesion to detect carcinoma or inflammatory bowel disease.

Blood loss from haemorrhoids is usually not severe enough to cause anaemia. Rectal bleeding with anaemia is more likely to be due to carcinoma, angiodysplasia or inflammatory bowel disease.

INVESTIGATING RECTAL BLEEDING

The majority of conditions can be diagnosed with a careful history and examination with proctoscopy and sigmoidoscopy. However, further investigation may be required if the diagnosis is equivocal:

- Full blood count is essential to establish whether anaemia is present.
- Colonoscopy or flexible sigmoidoscopy allow higher sigmoid lesions, and many vascular lesions such as angiodysplasia, to be seen. More than two-thirds of all colonic polyps and tumours occur within 60 cm of the anal margin.
- Angiography can be performed to locate the site of bleeding. Treatment by radiologically-guided embolization may be possible. Angiography tends to be useful only if there is active bleeding (at least 0.5 mL per minute).

Summary

An algorithm summarizing the investigation of rectal bleeding is shown in Fig. 10.1.

Fig. 10.1 Investigation of rectal bleeding.

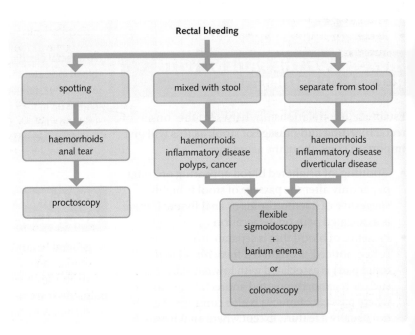

Anaemia is a low haemoglobin concentration in plasma, due to a low red cell mass. The symptoms of anaemia occur as a result of the reduced oxygen-carrying capacity of blood and therefore the reduced delivery of oxygen to tissues. Gastrointestinal causes of anaemia include:

- Reduced intake (e.g. dietary deficiencies of iron, folate and vitamin B_{12}).
- Reduced absorption (e.g. pernicious anaemia, small bowel disease such as Crohn's, coeliac disease or bacterial overgrowth, achlorhydria following gastrectomy).
- Gastrointestinal blood loss (e.g. from peptic ulcer disease, oesophagitis, occult carcinoma or angiodysplasia).

In a patient with iron-deficiency anaemia, don't forget to ask about other possible sources of blood loss. A patient would probably mention haematuria, but it is easy to forget heavy menstrual loss as a cause of anaemia. In fact, up to 25% of women younger than 45 years can be anaemic. This may help prevent unnecessary gastrointestinal investigations.

HISTORY OF THE PATIENT WITH ANAEMIA

Depending on the severity of anaemia and the presence of concurrent pathology, the patient can present with symptoms of anaemia such as:

- Fatigue.
- Palpitations.
- Shortness of breath.
- Angina pectoris.

Frequently, the detection of anaemia is an incidental finding on a routine blood test when the patient presents with unrelated symptoms.

The following aspects of the history should be considered in detail.

Symptoms of anaemia such as fatigue are thought to require a reduction in haemoglobin concentration of about 25%. For practical purposes, this means that symptoms are uncommon unless haemoglobin is <8 g/dL (females) or <10 g/dL (males).

Diet

Check whether the patient has a well-balanced diet:

- Meat contains haem iron, which is more readily bioavailable than non-haem iron.

- Fresh vegetables and fruit are important sources of the reductants (e.g. vitamin C) necessary to make iron bioavailable, resulting in the conversion of Fe^{3+} to Fe^{2+}.

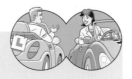

A dietary history is important to help assess for potential nutritional deficiencies.
Vegans are particularly at risk of iron and vitamin B_{12} deficiency. Recalling and describing usual food intake can be difficult, so asking a patient to keep a food diary for 7 days can be particularly helpful.

Past medical and surgical history

Clearly, previous surgical procedures may be pertinent, such as:

- Partial gastrectomy resulting in achlorhydria and thus preventing reduction of iron.
- Terminal ileal resection, leading to vitamin B_{12} malabsorption.

Previous medical history is important for similar reasons:

- Long-term antisecretory medication could theoretically precipitate anaemia if iron stores were already low.
- Crohn's disease or tuberculosis can affect terminal ileal absorption.
- Use of non-steroidal anti-inflammatory agents, including low-dose aspirin, is associated with chronic occult blood loss.

Associated features

Consider the following associated features:

- Diarrhoea with anaemia is a common manifestation of malabsorption. Chronic diarrhoea due to giardiasis or hookworm infestation is a common cause of anaemia worldwide. Coeliac disease is possibly the most common cause of malabsorption presenting with anaemia in the Western world.
- Anaemia due to chronic gastrointestinal (GI) blood loss may be associated with dyspeptic symptoms related to acid reflux or peptic ulcer

disease. Upper GI malignancy can present as anaemia.
- Haematemesis is not usually ignored by patients but melaena occasionally is.

Look for features of anaemia such as:

- Pallor.
- Tachycardia, or cardiac failure.

Pale conjunctivae correlate very poorly with haemoglobin concentration and cannot be relied upon as a sign.

Particular signs to look for include:

- Koilonychia (associated with iron deficiency).
- Atrophic glossitis (iron and vitamin B_{12} deficiency).
- Surgical scars (see Fig. 22.10) (e.g. midline scar of gastric surgery, previous ileal resection, etc.).
- Peri-oral pigmentation in Peutz–Jeghers syndrome (associated with GI polyps, particularly in the upper GI tract).
- Telangiectasia around the mouth and tongue (associated with hereditary haemorrhagic telangiectasia which can cause bleeding from the GI tract).
- Signs of chronic liver disease (See Ch. 18). Liver disease can be associated with anaemia:
  - Blood loss from varices or portal hypertensive gastropathy.
  - Zieve's syndrome (a type of haemolytic anaemia occurring in alcoholics).
- Splenomegaly (may indicate hypersplenism):
  - Hepatosplenomegaly in chronic liver disease.
  - Lymphoproliferative disorders.

Rectal examination is mandatory in iron deficiency:

- Rectal carcinoma.
- Confirm melaena (upper GI tract blood loss).
- Fresh blood on glove (lower GI blood loss).

INVESTIGATING ANAEMIA

The full blood count is necessary not only to confirm the presence of anaemia, but also as an important key to its subsequent investigation. The severity of the anaemia is determined by haemoglobin and haematocrit. Important clues to the aetiology are often given by the red blood cell size and haemoglobin content:

- A microcytic, hypochromic picture is due to iron deficiency. This can result from dietary deficiency, failure of absorption or blood loss. A blood film may demonstrate anisocytosis and poikilocytosis (variation in size and shape of the red cell, respectively).
- A normocytic, normochromic picture is commonly associated with chronic inflammatory disease, in which iron stores are adequate but not utilized effectively.
- A macrocytic picture can be due to folate or vitamin B_{12} deficiency, alcohol, hypothyroidism or certain drugs (e.g. phenytoin—antifolate action), or hydroxyurea.

Further investigation, therefore, is dependent on the full blood count indices.

If macrocytic anaemia is due to vitamin B_{12} deficiency because of bacterial overgrowth, serum folate will be elevated as a consequence of bacterial metabolism. Otherwise, folate is often also deficient.

Biochemistry

Biochemistry tests may aid diagnosis (Fig. 11.1):

- Serum ferritin is the most sensitive test to reflect iron stores, but, as an 'acute phase protein', it may be falsely elevated in the presence of a concomitant inflammatory condition.
- Serum folate should be measured in any patient with macrocytosis. Deficiency is usually due to malabsorption (most commonly coeliac disease), poor dietary intake, excessive use as in pregnancy or increased cell turnover in malignancy or red cell haemolysis. Antifolate drugs, such as methotrexate, and antibiotics, such as trimethoprim, also cause folate deficiency.

Fig.11.1 Parameters to differentiate iron-deficiency anaemia from anaemia of chronic disease

	Anaemia of chronic disease	Iron deficiency
MCV	↓/normal	↓
Serum iron	↓	↓
TIBC	↓	↑
Ferritin	↓/normal/↑	↓
Iron stores in bone marrow (Perl's stain)	normal	↓/absent
Iron in red-cell precursors	↓	↓/absent

(MCV, mean cell volume; TIBC, total iron-binding capacity.)

- Vitamin B_{12} must also be measured in patients with macrocytosis. If deficient, a Schilling test (see Ch. 24) may be helpful in deciding the cause.
- Blood urea can be useful. It is often raised following an upper GI bleed which is effectively a large protein meal. Dehydration may also contribute.
- Faeces can be tested for occult blood loss, although both false positive and false negative results can be obtained.

Endoscopy

Gastroscopy should be undertaken in all cases of iron-deficiency anaemia, unless there is clearly an alternative explanation, to exclude oesophagitis, gastric ulcer or erosions, and carcinoma.

The presence of a duodenal ulcer is an insufficient explanation for iron-deficiency anaemia. A biopsy of the second part of the duodenum should be taken at the same time, to exclude coeliac disease.

Colonoscopy is the preferred large bowel investigation because it should identify all lesions resulting in blood loss, including angiodysplasia. When it is not practical, barium examination should be undertaken.

Radiology

A barium meal is indicated if there is suspicion of gastric carcinoma and gastroscopy is not possible. Similarly, a barium enema will demonstrate the presence of diverticular disease, polyps and carcinoma, but endoscopy is preferable in order to ascribe the cause of bleeding to a particular lesion or to identify angiodysplasia.

Angiography is helpful in the presence of active bleeding, but is not generally rewarding in the investigation of chronic anaemia.

Other tests for anaemia

Other tests may be useful:

- A Schilling test may help differentiate the different causes of vitamin B_{12} deficiency (see Ch. 24).
- A ^{14}C-glycocholic acid breath test or a lactulose hydrogen breath test may be used to investigate bacterial overgrowth (see Ch. 24).

- A ^{99}Tc radio-isotope scan is helpful if a Meckel's diverticulum is suspected of causing chronic anaemia in a young patient.
- A ^{51}Cr-labelled red cell scan may give a clue to the general location of occult blood loss, but is not helpful to identify the nature of the lesion or the precise anatomical location.
- A chest X-ray is mandatory in a smoker with unexplained anaemia to exclude lung cancer.
- Consider serum electrophoresis and testing urine for Bence–Jones protein to exclude myeloma in a patient with unexplained normocytic anaemia.

Summary

An algorithm summarizing the investigation of anaemia is given in Fig. 11.2.

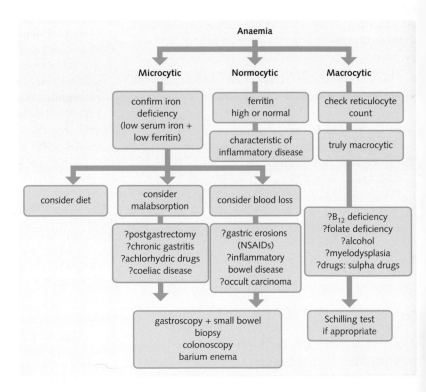

Fig. 11.2 Algorithm for the gastrointestinal investigation of anaemia. (NSAIDs, non-steroidal anti-inflammatory drugs.)

Jaundice 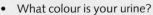 12

Objectives

You should be able to:

- Take a history from a jaundiced patient
- Describe and classify the causes of jaundice
- Understand how to distinguish between pre-hepatic, hepatic and post-hepatic jaundice
- Describe the clinical findings in chronic liver disease

Jaundice is a yellow colouring of the skin and sclerae due to elevated levels of bilirubin in plasma. Jaundice is usually clinically evident if serum bilirubin exceeds 40 μmol/L (about twice the normal upper limit). There are numerous causes of jaundice and a careful history and examination are vital so that unnecessary invasive investigations can be avoided.

The more common causes include:

- Haemolytic anaemias or ineffective erythropoiesis such as autoimmune haemolytic anaemia or haemoglobinopathies, respectively.
- Congenital hyperbilirubinaemia due to enzyme defects, most commonly Gilbert's syndrome.
- Extra-hepatic bile duct obstruction due to gallstones, pancreatitis or pancreatic cancer.
- Sclerosing cholangitis.
- Intra-hepatic cholestasis due to drugs, alcohol, hepatitis or chronic liver disease.

HISTORY OF THE PATIENT WITH JAUNDICE

All aspects of the history should be taken with care as there are times when certain facts can appear to be trivial, yet may later become vital in the diagnosis. The following features help to differentiate causes of jaundice (Fig. 12.1).

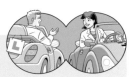

The key questions to ask a patient with jaundice are:
- What colour is your urine?
- What colour are your stools?
  Dark urine and pale stools signify cholestasis (failure of bile to flow from the liver). These questions separate pre-hepatic jaundice (acholuric jaundice) from the other varieties (hepatic and post-hepatic).
  An ultrasound scan will separate hepatic and post-hepatic jaundice. If it shows dilated biliary ducts, then this implies obstruction (e.g. from gallstones) as the cause of the cholestasis.

Age

Younger patients are more likely to have congenital hyperbilirubinaemia or viral hepatitis than carcinoma of the pancreas, which rarely affects those aged less than 60 years.

Onset of symptoms

The onset of symptoms may give clues to the diagnosis:

- An acute onset is more likely to be of infective or drug-induced aetiology.
- A slow insidious onset is more likely to be due to chronic active hepatitis (e.g. caused by autoimmune disease or alcohol).

Fig. 12.1 Causes of jaundice

	Causes of jaundice	Drugs
Pre-hepatic	• haemolysis • ineffective erythropoiesis • Gilbert's and Crigler–Najjar syndromes	

Hepatic	• viruses: Hep A, B, C, E
	      Epstein–Barr
	      cytomegalovirus
	      herpes simplex/zoster
	• leptospirosis/toxoplasmosis
	• autoimmune hepatitis
	• cirrhosis
	• Wilson's disease
	• rotor/Dubin–Johnson syndrome
		• isoniazid
		• paracetamol excess
		• chlorpromazine

Post-hepatic	• intra-hepatic: primary biliary cirrhosis
	      primary sclerosing
	      cholangitis
	      cholangiocarcinoma
	      +same causes listed
	      under Hepatic
	• extra-hepatic: gallstones
	      carcinoma of head of
	      pancreas
	      enlarged lymph nodes
	      at porta hepatis
		Drugs causing cholestasis:
		• oral contraceptive pill
		• flucloxacillin
		  or co-amoxiclav
		• anabolic steroids

Infectious contact and risk behaviour

It is important to establish whether the patient has any risk factors for developing jaundice:

- Find out whether there has been contact with other people with jaundice, such as occurs in epidemics of hepatitis A and E or infectious mononucleosis (Epstein–Barr virus).
- Has there been high-risk behaviour for exposure to hepatitis B (promiscuous sexual activity or shared needles)?
- A history of recent travel abroad is also essential: ingestion of seafood abroad is a common source of infectious hepatitis. Do not forget exotic causes such as yellow fever from Africa!
- Occupational or recreational history may be relevant: sewage and farm workers are at risk of leptospirosis, as well as windsurfers and people who go pot-holing.
- A history of excess alcohol consumption must be excluded and tactful discussion with relatives may be necessary.

Past medical history

This may immediately suggest a diagnosis. For example:

- Previous cholecystectomy could suggest a bile duct stone or stricture.
- Ulcerative colitis can predispose to sclerosing cholangitis in 3–6%.

Patients often forget that they have had antibiotics or other drugs recently and liaison with their general practitioner may be helpful.

Drugs

Many drugs are metabolized in the liver, and some cause idiosyncratic reactions, resulting in jaundice. Others have a dose-related effect, resulting in liver damage and jaundice. Important drugs to consider include:

- Antibiotics such as co-amoxiclav or flucloxacillin.
- Antifungal agents such as fluconazole.
- Allopurinol which can occasionally cause profound jaundice.

- Antituberculous drugs such as isoniazid or rifampicin.
- Neuroleptics such as chlorpromazine.
- Paracetamol in excess of therapeutic dose.

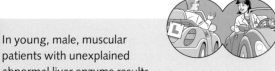

In young, male, muscular patients with unexplained abnormal liver enzyme results, it can be revealing to ask about illicit use of anabolic steroids. They may have cholestasis as a result of the drug itself, but individuals are also at risk of hepatitis B and C from contaminated needles.

Family history

A history of intermittent jaundice in the family suggests congenital hyperbilirubinaemia. Also enquire about Wilson's disease and alpha-1-antitrypsin deficiency.

Associated features

A number of features may suggest underlying pathology, such as:

- Presence of abdominal pain, particularly if localized to the right upper quadrant—suggests bile duct stones or pain originating from the liver capsule.
- Acute onset abdominal distension with jaundice—may indicate acute hepatitis or hepatic vein thrombosis (resulting in ascites).
- Painless jaundice in conjunction with weight loss in older patients—suggestive of carcinoma of the pancreas or enlarged metastatic lymph nodes at the porta hepatis.
- Signs of cardiac failure, especially elevated jugular venous pressure and peripheral oedema—may indicate a congested liver with jaundice.

EXAMINING THE PATIENT WITH JAUNDICE

Assess the severity of the jaundice clinically:

- Acute jaundice has a bright yellow hue.

- Chronic jaundice has a dusky appearance and, if severe, the patient may look green.

Look for signs of anaemia, which may indicate underlying haemolysis.

Generalized lymphadenopathy may be due to Epstein–Barr, cytomegalovirus (CMV) or toxoplasmosis.

Check for features of chronic liver disease or cirrhosis (see Ch. 18), such as:

- Parotitis.
- Spider naevi.
- Gynaecomastia and loss of secondary sexual characterisitics.
- Palmar erythema.
- Splenomegaly (think of infections, haemolysis or portal hypertension).
- Hepatomegaly.
- Ascites (may be acute in Budd–Chiari syndrome).

Kayser–Fleischer rings are present in 70% of patients with Wilson's disease. They are seen as a brown ring in the periphery of the cornea, most often at the top. Slit lamp examination may be necessary.

The gall bladder may be palpated in a patient with progressive, painless jaundice due to obstruction. If, in painless jaundice, the gall bladder is palpable, the cause will not be gallstones (Courvoisier's law). In elderly patients, this is commonly due to carcinoma of the head of the pancreas.

Associated systemic signs may suggest particular syndromes with liver involvement:

- Chronic respiratory disease with jaundice may occur with cystic fibrosis or alpha-1-antitrypsin deficiency.
- Neurological signs, particular those of parkinsonism, with jaundice may suggest hepatolenticular degeneration (Wilson's disease).

INVESTIGATING JAUNDICE

Abdominal ultrasound is the key investigation in a patient with jaundice because it will differentiate obstructive jaundice from other causes, and the subsequent approaches to management are different. If the bile ducts are not dilated, then blood tests become useful to differentiate causes of jaundice:

- Urine testing for bilirubin and urobilinogen is an inexpensive and useful test to investigate the potential aetiologies. Unconjugated jaundice (e.g. Gilbert's or haemolysis) will result in an absence of bilirubin in the urine. Biliary obstruction will demonstrate increased urinary bilirubin and absent or reduced urobilinogen. If there is active red cell haemolysis, then urinary haemosiderin may be detectable.
- The pattern of abnormalities in liver enzymes and other associated blood tests help indicate the cause of jaundice (see Ch. 13).

Prothrombin time is influenced by vitamin K, as this is a required co-factor for coagulation factors II, VII, IX and X. Because vitamin K is a fat-soluble vitamin, its absorption is reduced in biliary duct obstruction, when sufficient bile fails to reach the small intestine. In this situation, a single dose of intravenous vitamin K may correct the prothrombin time; it will have no effect if the coagulopathy is due to deficient synthesis of coagulation factors, as in parenchymal liver diseases.

- Percutaneous liver biopsy can provide valuable information regarding both the cause and extent of parenchymal liver damage. It is usually performed under ultrasound guidance, and the prothrombin time must be checked pre biopsy. Special staining for copper and alpha-1-antitrypsin can be performed on histological sections.
- A computed tomography scan of the abdomen is mainly used to assess pancreatic masses and nodes at the porta hepatis when obstructive jaundice has been confirmed by ultrasound.
- Magnetic resonance cholangiography or endoscopic ultrasound are useful examinations for assessment of the bile duct, while obviating the serious risk of acute pancreatitis which exists with an endoscopic retrograde cholangiopancreatography.
- Endoscopic retrograde cholangiopancreatography or percutaneous transhepatic cholangiography is useful for therapy if there is obstructive jaundice (e.g. removal of gallstones, insertion of a biliary stent).

Summary

An algorithm summarizing the investigation of a patient with jaundice is shown in Fig. 12.2.

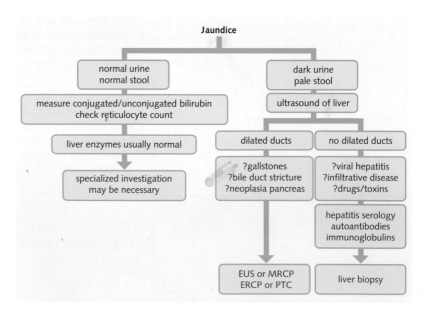

Fig. 12.2 Algorithm for the investigation of a patient with jaundice. (ERCP, endoscopic retrograde cholangiopancreatography; EUS, endoscopic ultrasound; MRCP, magnetic resonance cholangiopancreatography; PTC, percutaneous transhepatic cholangiography.)

Abnormal liver biochemistry

Objectives

You should be able to:

- Take a history from a patient with abnormal liver biochemistry
- Distinguish between a cholestatic and hepatitic pattern of abnormalities of liver biochemistry

Patients are commonly referred to the gastroenterology clinic for investigation of abnormal liver biochemistry. This may have been detected while investigating pertinent symptoms, or discovered incidentally during investigation of other complaints. The four enzymes involved are:

- Alanine aminotransferase (ALT or SGPT in older texts).
- Aspartate aminotransferase (AST or SGOT in older texts).
- Alkaline phosphatase (AlkPhos).
- Gamma-glutamyl transferase (GGT).

Often these tests are referred to as liver 'function' tests. This is misleading because the elevation of liver enzymes does not reflect hepatic function.

Abnormal liver enzymes in the absence of jaundice may be commonly due to:

- Acute or chronic liver disease.
- Cirrhosis.
- Drugs, including alcohol.
- Liver metastasis.
- Cardiac causes such as acute myocardial infarction, cardiac failure and constrictive pericarditis.
- Hypothyroidism or pernicious anaemia—occasionally present with elevated transaminases.
- Severe sepsis or atypical pneumonias—can result in deranged liver enzymes.
  Alkaline phosphatase will be increased in:
- Bone disease (e.g. Paget's, bony metastases; unchanged in osteoporosis).
- Pregnancy.

- Acute inflammatory response.
- Young adults or children (bones are still growing).

HISTORY OF THE PATIENT WITH ABNORMAL LIVER BIOCHEMISTRY

It is first essential to establish the chronology of the abnormalities. When were the results last normal? Assess the trend of abnormalities and attempt to correlate this with relevant drug interventions and medical history.

Patients are usually asymptomatic when referred to outpatient clinics, or tests may have been carried out for vague symptoms such as malaise or fatigue. Hence it is important to interpret the results in context, in order to focus appropriate investigation and avoid further unnecessary tests.

The following points usually help.

Drug history

Prescribed medication is one of the most common cause of abnormal liver biochemistry in the general population, apart from alcohol:

- Antibiotics such as flucloxacillin or co-amoxiclav can result in elevated transaminases, that can remain elevated for several weeks after their cessation. They can also cause jaundice.
- Many anti-arthritis drugs and anti-epileptic drugs (such as phenytoin or carbamazepine) can induce liver enzymes.

An accurate drug history is essential in the investigation of unexplained abnormal liver enzymes and it may be helpful to telephone the GP to establish the date that prescriptions have been issued. Patients may not mention over-the-counter medicines. Some herbal medications can have profound effects on liver enzymes or may interact with other drugs the patient may be taking.

Alcohol

Alcohol is often the first thing that comes to mind in relation to liver disease. However, as an aetiological agent, it accounts for less than 20% of patients with liver disease attending outpatients.

There is no specific pattern to liver enzymes with alcohol use:

- GGT is easily induced and the most common liver abnormality to be seen.
- As an isolated abnormality, GGT is of little significance; its most useful role is indicating that a raised AlkPhos is of liver origin.
- An AST to ALT ratio of 2 or more is said to be specific for alcoholic hepatitis, but it is not a sensitive indicator.

Past medical history and surgical history

A history of biliary tract surgery, including cholecystectomy, is particularly relevant. Otherwise, history should concentrate on those aspects discussed in Ch. 12.

EXAMINING THE PATIENT WITH ABNORMAL LIVER BIOCHEMISTRY

A general physical examination is clearly important, but, in particular, signs of liver disease should be sought as discussed in Ch. 12. Other medical conditions can also be associated with raised liver enzymes:

- Hypothyroidism.
- Pernicious anaemia.
- Congestive cardiac failure.
- Lymphoma.
- Diabetes mellitus or hypercholesterolaemia.
- Obesity.

INVESTIGATING ABNORMAL LIVER BIOCHEMISTRY

The investigation largely depends on the pattern of abnormality produced by the elevated enzymes. The following is simply intended as a guide and in clinical practice often it is difficult (sometimes impossible) to decipher the 'picture' of abnormality presented.

Drug-induced abnormalities do not require further investigation if, following cessation of the offending drug (including reducing alcohol intake), the biochemistry returns to normal within 8–12 weeks.

Liver chemistry tests

These tests may aid diagnosis:

- If at least three liver enzymes are raised, this would imply that significant liver pathology is present.
- A predominantly hepatitic abnormality is suggested if AST, ALT and, to a lesser extent, GGT are the most prominently raised enzymes. These may be only slightly elevated in certain conditions such as hepatitis C, haemochromatosis or alpha-1-antitrypsin deficiency.
- A predominantly cholestatic abnormality is suggested by raised AlkPhos and GGT with or without elevation of serum bilirubin. In this situation, think of intra-hepatic or extra-hepatic cholestasis. The most common causes in the absence of jaundice are drugs, cholangitis and primary biliary cirrhosis. Antimitochondrial antibodies may be helpful.
- Serum bilirubin does not necessarily reflect the degree of liver damage, particularly in the

acute situation. In chronic liver disease, it gives a reasonable indication of the stage of progression.

- Elevated bilirubin, but normal liver enzymes, indicates haemolysis, or a genetic defect in conjugation (Gilbert's syndrome, Crigler–Najjar syndrome) or export (Dubin–Johnson syndrome, Rotor syndrome) of bilirubin.

Other blood tests

The following may help direct further investigation:

- Full blood count may demonstrate macrocytosis, which in association with an elevated GGT implies alcohol as a causative factor. Thrombocytopaenia may indicate hypersplenism due to portal hypertension and cirrhosis.
- Hepatitis virus serology (see Ch. 18) is necessary, especially if ALT and AST (with or without an elevation of bilirubin) are primarily affected. Markers for leptospirosis should also be done if clinically indicated.
- An autoantibody screen may be appropriate if the demographics of the patient and the clinical picture are suggestive of autoimmune disease (see Ch. 18).
- Immunoglobulins—elevated immunoglobulin (Ig)A can be associated with alcohol-mediated damage. Raised IgM can indicate primary biliary cirrhosis and IgG is associated with chronic active hepatitis.
- Prothrombin time is the most easily available test that gives some indication of hepatic synthetic function, because all of the clotting factors are made in the liver. It correlates well with outcome in acute liver failure.
- Albumin, also synthesized in the liver, is reduced in any 'sick' state and correlates less well with severity of liver dysfunction. Similarly, blood urea is usually low but not very informative.

Dynamic and metabolic liver function tests

See Chapter 24.

Imaging

Ultrasound of the liver is essential to exclude bile duct dilatation, liver metastasis or other focal abnormality and hepatic congestion.

Cirrhosis is a histological diagnosis which cannot be made on ultrasound scanning alone, although there are features such as irregular margins and nodules that may suggest the diagnosis. Metastatic disease is occasionally confused with cirrhosis on ultrasound scans.

Biopsy

Liver biopsy may be necessary if no other explanation is found for the abnormal liver biochemistry. It can also be performed to establish the underlying cause of cirrhosis if suspected on ultrasound. Be sure to measure the prothrombin time first!

Exceptions to consider

Note the following:

- Raised GGT alone is highly suggestive of alcohol consumption or drugs that induce hepatic enzymes such as anticonvulsants; hence, further investigation is usually unnecessary.
- Raised AlkPhos alone may suggest a non-hepatic origin, such as bone, placenta or, very occasionally, intestine. Isoenzymes can be measured if necessary, to establish the origin.
- AST is also produced by heart and striated muscle. It can be raised in myocardial infarction, hypothyroidism and pernicious anaemia, hence its sole elevation should alert one to other medical conditions.
- ALT is much more specific for liver disease. A minor elevation on its own is probably of no consequence but, if raised in association with AlkPhos, it is usually an indication for further investigation including liver biopsy.
- There is no correlation between liver enzyme abnormalities and the extent of cirrhosis. The enzymes may be entirely normal even in advanced cirrhosis.

Summary

An algorithm summarizing the investigation of a patient referred with abnormal liver enzymes is shown in Fig. 13.1.

Other features include:

- Weight loss—consequent upon anorexia, dysphagia and possibly mediated by release of tumour cytokines.
- Anaemia due to ulceration of the lesion is common, and may cause insidious blood loss, resulting in iron-deficiency anaemia.
- Pain on swallowing (odynophagia) —occurs in advanced stages; local infiltration by the tumour causes diffuse and persistent retrosternal pain.
- Dyspnoea and cough—due to aspiration of pharyngeal secretions. In advanced cases, this may be due to oesophago-tracheal fistulae or tracheal encasement.

Diagnosis and investigation

Consider the following investigations:

- Full blood count may demonstrate iron-deficiency anaemia or rarely pancytopenia from metastatic bone marrow infiltration by tumour.
- Derangement of liver biochemistry or hypercalcaemia may be seen if metastases are present.
- Urea and electrolytes often reveal dehydration, as a result of dysphagia.
- Endoscopy—the investigation of choice because it allows direct visualization of the lesion and an opportunity for biopsy and histological confirmation.
- Barium swallow—reserved for patients who cannot tolerate an endoscopy, or those suspected of having a high-level stricture. Malignant strictures characteristically have a shouldered appearance (see Fig. 2.3B).
- Endoscopic ultrasound and spiral computed tomography (CT) scan of thorax—used for staging of disease.
- Positron emission tomography (PET) scans and combined CT/PET scanning is being used (where available) to aid staging in early disease.

Aetiology and pathogenesis

Rarely occurs under the age of 50 years. Two histological types are seen:

- Squamous carcinoma.
- Adenocarcinoma.

Squamous carcinoma:

- Ninety per cent of all oesophageal cancer is squamous in nature.

- Fifty per cent of all squamous cancers occur in the lower third of the oesophagus.
- Higher incidence in China, which may suggest a dietary aetiology.
- More common in men, particularly with high alcohol intake and cigarette smoking.
- More unusual predisposing factors include achalasia, Plummer–Vinson syndrome and tylosis (hyperkeratosis of the palms and soles inherited as a rare autosomal dominant condition).

Adenocarcinoma:

- Usually as a result of malignant transformation of Barrett's oesophagus.
- Occasionally, it arises as an extension from adenocarcinoma of gastric cardia.

Complications

The tumour may invade adjacent anatomical structures:

- Through the oesophageal wall and into a bronchus, creating an oesophageal–bronchial fistula, resulting in recurrent pneumonia (note that aspiration pneumonia may occur as a result of severe dysphagia in the absence of a fistula).
- Into the thoracic aorta, resulting in rapid exsanguination.

Prognosis

To some extent, this is dependent on stage of the tumour and fitness of the patient. However, the prognosis is usually exceptionally poor, with an overall survival of 2% at 5 years.

Treatment

Treatment is mainly palliative because curative treatment is rarely possible due to late presentation of the disease. Consider:

- Surgery—provides the only possible cure but carries an operative mortality of 5–10%. Less than 40% of patients are suitable for surgical resection at presentation, but these patients are often elderly and frail with medical co-morbidity precluding radical surgery.
- Radiotherapy—reduces the bulk of the tumour and may relieve dysphagia. Fistula formation is more common after radiotherapy treatment.

- Laser therapy—high-energy thermal laser ablation is used to burn through the bulk of the tumour and restore the oesophageal lumen. An alternative for smaller tumours is photodynamic therapy, using a lower energy laser light in combination with a chemical photosensitizer which is selectively taken up by tumour tissue. Repeated administration of either modality may be required.
- Endoscopic placement of an expanding metal hollow stent (endoprosthesis) across the obstructing lesion can give palliative relief of dysphagia. This carries a risk of perforation in up to 10% of patients.
- Brachytherapy (local radiotherapy applied by placement of radioactive implants at the tumour site) has been used for palliation.

Cases are considered by a multidisciplinary team (surgeon, gastroenterologist, pathologist, radiologist, oncologist, dietician, specialist nurses, etc.).

Tumour-node metastasis (TNM) classification of tumours

The approach to management of many malignant tumours depends on their stage. In addition, a comparison of treatment strategies is heavily reliant on making sure that like is compared with like.

An internationally accepted classification for tumours is the TNM staging system. This system varies for different organs and tissues but follows the general principle shown in Fig. 14.4:

- 'T' refers to the extent of the tumour itself: T0 usually indicates no detectable tumour, T1 is confined to mucosa, and T3+ is infiltrating deeper layers or surrounding structures depending on the site.
- Similarly, 'N' refers to lymph node involvement: N0 means no node involvement, N1 is usually confined to local nodes and N2+ is confined to more distant nodes specified for that tumour type.
- Very distant nodes are usually classified as 'M' for metastatic: M0 means no metastases detected, Mn indicates distant spread, again 'n' having a specific meaning for each tumour type.

Thus, T4N2M2 is a tumour with:

- Extensive local infiltration.
- Distant lymph node involvement.
- Metastatic spread to other sites.

Pharyngeal pouch and oesophageal diverticulum

Incidence

Usually discovered coincidentally while a barium meal is performed for other reasons.

Clinical features

The majority are asymptomatic, although they can cause regurgitation of food and are a rare cause of dysphagia.

Diagnosis and investigation

Barium swallow demonstrates the size and location of the lesion (Fig. 14.5).

Aetiology and pathogenesis

Probably related to dysmotility of cricopharyngeus muscle and inferior constrictor forming a mucosal outpouching (pharyngeal pouch). Diverticulae may also occur in the mid oesophagus due to traction by mediastinal lymph node inflammation (traction diverticulum), or just above the lower oesophageal sphincter (epiphrenic diverticulum).

Complications

Occur rarely—perforation may occur when endoscopy is performed for investigation of dysphagia, as the pouch may be mistaken for the oesophageal lumen!

Treatment

Surgical resection is reserved for pouches that are problematic.

Oesophageal web

Incidence

Oesophageal web is often a coincidental finding on barium meal. Those associated with iron-deficiency anaemia are rare.

Clinical features

Usually the patient is asymptomatic, but high-level dysphagia may occur when tough fibrous food is

Fig. 14.4 Graphic illustration of the tumour-node metastasis (TNM) classification of mucosal malignant disease. T0, no evidence of primary tumour; T1, tumour confined to mucosa; T2, infiltration through sub mucosa but not penetrating through the muscularis; T3, extends through muscularis to serosa; T4, extends to local tissues; N0, no lymph node involvement; N1, local lymph node involvement; N2, distant lymph node involvement.

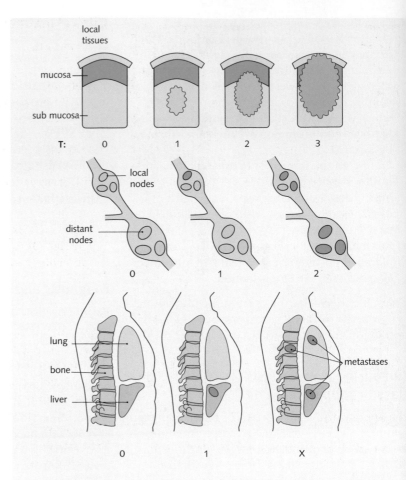

T = graded 0–4, refers to the primary tumour according to its depth of involvement
T0 = no evidence of primary tumour

N = 0–2, refers to lymph nodes involved; increasing score indicates higher numbers of lymph node involvment

M = 0 or 1 refers to presence and absence of metastases. The example shown might be for carcinoma of the colon

swallowed without care. There may be a history of a persistent cough, due to the aspiration of pharyngeal secretions.

Anaemia may present as part of the Plummer–Vinson syndrome (see below).

Diagnosis and investigation

- Barium swallow—demonstrates narrowing of the oesophagus by fibrous tissue. The proximal part of the oesophagus may be distended with barium.
- Endoscopy—webs may be difficult to see, especially those in the postcricoid area.

Aetiology and pathogenesis

Unknown aetiology—different clinical outcome depending on site of the web. Two types are commonly recognized:

- Postcricoid web.
- Lower oesophageal web.

Postcricoid web:

- Is also know as Plummer–Vinson or Paterson–Brown–Kelly syndrome.
- Is associated with iron deficiency anaemia and atrophic glossitis.

Clinical features

These include:

- Intermittent dysphagia—usually a long history with both liquids and solids. Presentation in childhood is rare.
- Regurgitation—common; may result in aspiration pneumonia if it occurs at night-time. Dysphagia can sometimes be overcome by drinking large quantities of fluid; hence, increases risk of aspiration.
- Chest pain—this is common and is typically retrosternal and occasionally severe, due to non-peristaltic contraction of the oesophageal muscles. Often mistaken for cardiac pain, especially when dysphagic symptoms are mild.

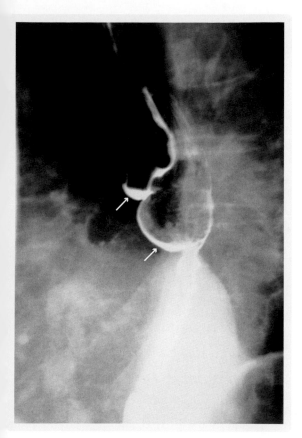

Fig. 14.5 Lateral view of oesophageal diverticulum (arrows) in the upper oesophagus seen on barium swallow. Note the fluid levels.

Lower oesophageal web:

- Is also known as a Schatzki ring, where there is a small, fibromuscular band that originates from the diaphragm.
- Is often associated with a hiatus hernia.

Patients may appear to have achalasia on the basis on radiological and endoscopic findings. However, the term 'pseudoachalasia' is used to describe conditions that mimic achalasia, for example small cancers. Ask the patient how fast their symptoms appeared and whether they have had weight loss. Rapid onset symptoms, weight loss or any older patient with achalasia-like symptoms may benefit from other tests (CT scan or endoscopic ultrasound scan) to exclude more serious disease.

Complications

There is an increased risk of developing postcricoid carcinoma of the pharynx associated with Plummer–Vinson syndrome.

Treatment

Dilatation of the obstruction is rarely needed.

Oral iron supplementation may be required if iron-deficiency anaemia, associated with Plummer–Vinson syndrome, is present.

Achalasia

Incidence

Achalasia is a rare condition with an incidence of approximately 1:100 000 per year.

Diagnosis and investigation

The following investigations should be considered:

- Chest X-ray—may show a double cardiac shadow with a fluid level behind the heart. Evidence of pneumonia, or atelectasis implying previous infection, may also be present. Aspiration classically occurs down the right main bronchus, into the right middle and lower lobes.
- Barium swallow—dilatation of the oesophagus is seen with a narrowed lower portion (beak appearance) due to lack of relaxation by the lower oesophageal sphincter (Fig. 14.6). Reduced peristaltic contraction is also seen.

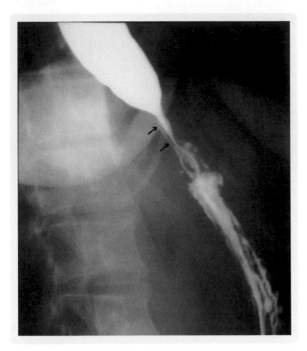

Fig. 14.6 Barium swallow showing 'bird's beak' appearance of achalasia.

- Endoscopy—the scope usually passes through the narrowed region without resistance, and is therefore often missed. Sometimes there is some resistance to the passage of the scope (the positive 'tug' sign).
- Motility studies—used to confirm lack of peristalsis along the oesophagus and failure of relaxation by the lower oesophageal sphincter (see Fig. 24.10B).
- Endoscopic ultrasound—may be helpful in excluding submucosal malignant infiltration and can show characteristic muscle thickening.

Aetiology and pathogenesis

Unknown aetiology—characterized by lack of peristalsis and failure of relaxation by the lower oesophageal sphincter (LOS) after swallowing.

Histology shows a reduction of Auerbach plexus ganglia cells in the oesophageal walls.

Infection with *Trypanosoma cruzi* (Chagas' disease or American trypanosomiasis) will produce a similar disorder.

Complications and prognosis

- There is an increased risk of developing oesophageal carcinoma (up to 10% higher than the normal population).

- Reflux oesophagitis is a major complication after treatment.

Treatment

Treatment may include:

- Dilatation with high-pressure balloons—this is undertaken endoscopically and is successful in over two-thirds of cases. It is accompanied by perforation in approximately 3–4%.
- Surgical division of muscle fibres at the lower end of the oesophagus (cardiomyotomy)—can now be performed laparoscopically.
- Calcium antagonists (e.g. nifedipine)—reduce LOS pressure and may be used by elderly patients who are unsuitable for procedures. Ten per cent of patients will benefit.
- Botulinum toxin may be injected into the LOS. Its duration of action is usually limited to only a few months and repeat treatments may be given.

Oesophageal spasm

Clinical features

Chest pain is retrosternal and severe, and often radiates to the back. It can be relieved by nitrates; hence, it is difficult to distinguish from ischaemic cardiac pain.

Dysphagia can occur due to marked contraction of oesophageal muscles.

Diagnosis and investigation

The following investigations may be used:

- Barium swallow—characteristically demonstrates a 'corkscrew' appearance due to uncoordinated contraction of the oesophageal muscles (see Fig. 1.5). However, similar changes may be seen in elderly people without any symptoms.
- Motility studies—show diffuse contraction of the oesophageal muscles without progression of peristalsis. Pressures can be very high ('nutcracker' oesophagus).

Aetiology and pathogenesis

Unknown aetiology—after swallowing, the oesophagus contracts diffusely in an uncoordinated fashion without peristalsis; hence the onset of dysphagia and chest pain.

Complications

Formation of diverticula is commonly associated with oesophageal dysmotility. Cricopharyngeal spasm is closely related to formation of pharyngeal pouches.

Treatment

Drugs such as antispasmodics, calcium channel antagonists or nitrates may be of help. Surgery, such as myotomy, may be required in exceptional cases.

Stomach

Objectives

You should be able to:

- Understand the main physiological functions of the stomach
- Describe investigations that can be employed to detect the presence of *Helicobacter pylori*
- Understand how non-steroidal anti-inflammatory drugs (NSAIDs) predispose toward peptic ulceration
- Describe the mechanism of action of proton pump inhibitors and H$_2$ antagonists
- Describe how you would manage a patient in the first few hours following an acute upper gastrointestinal bleed
- Understand the mechanisms by which anaemia may occur after gastrectomy

ANATOMY, PHYSIOLOGY AND FUNCTION OF THE STOMACH

The stomach is divided into:

An upper portion known as the fundus.
The body of the stomach.
The antrum, which extends to form the pyloric region, encompassing the pyloric sphincter (Fig. 15.1).

Three muscle layers form the stomach: outer longitudinal, middle circular and inner oblique. The thickened circular layer at the pyloric area forms the pyloric sphincter.

The upper two-thirds of the stomach contains:

Parietal cells which secrete acid (hydrochloric acid) and intrinsic factor.
Chief cells which secrete pepsinogen.

The antrum secretes gastrin from G cells which stimulates acid production.

Acid secretion consists of three different phases (Fig. 15.2):

Cephalic—mediated via the vagus, stimulated by sight or smell of food.
Gastric distension of the stomach by food directly stimulates secretory cells.

- Intestinal hormones are released as food is passed into the small intestine, stimulating acid release.

A low pH in the stomach is required to activate enzymes required for digestion and to act as a barrier

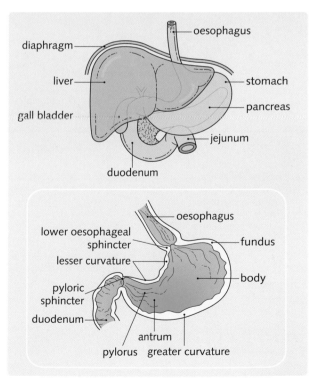

Fig. 15.1 Anatomical relations of the stomach.

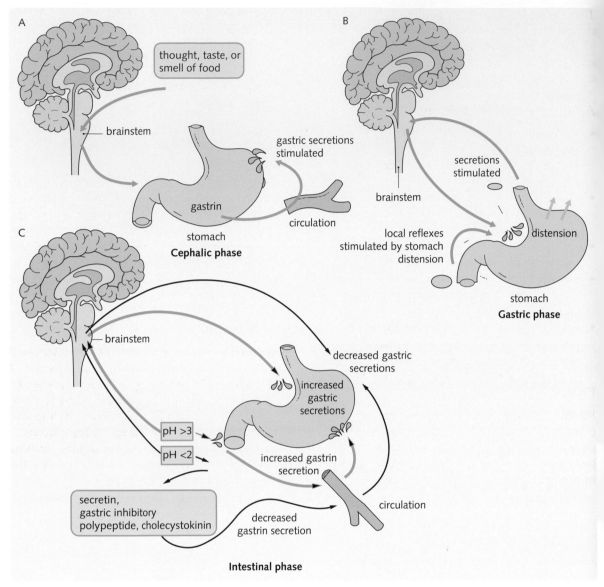

Fig. 15.2 Physiology of acid secretion. (A) Cephalic phase in which taste, visual and olfactory senses act through the brainstem and parasympathetic system to cause gastrin secretion, which in turn stimulates acid production. (B) Gastric phase in which ingested food distends the stomach and stretch receptors act through brainstem reflexes to increase gastric secretions. (C) Food in the intestine has different effects depending upon the pH. At higher pH, the pathways are stimulatory and increase gastric secretion further (green lines); at lower pH, negative and inhibitory factors come into play to reduce gastric secretion (black lines).

to bacteria. Other functions of the stomach include absorption of glucose and amino acids.

ACUTE GASTRITIS

Incidence

A very common condition with a variety of causes.

Clinical features

- Dyspepsia, nausea and vomiting are the most likely presenting symptoms.
- Acute gastrointestinal (GI) bleed if gastritis is severe.
- Asymptomatic.

Diagnosis and investigation

The diagnosis is often made on clinical grounds (e.g. history of NSAIDs), heavy alcohol consumption, etc.

There may be epigastric tenderness but this is not a discriminating sign.

Endoscopic appearance can vary from superficial erosions to haemorrhage secondary to acute ulceration.

Aetiology and pathogenesis

- The pathological appearance is that of an acute inflammatory infiltrate in the superficial mucosa, predominantly of neutrophils. Occasionally, superficial ulceration can be seen.
- Drugs such as aspirin and other NSAIDs reduce the production of prostaglandin and interfere with cytoprotection.
- Alcohol damages the mucosal mucus layer and causes gastritis.
- *Helicobacter pylori* can also cause acute gastritis, but is more commonly associated with chronic gastritis.
- Acute illness (sepsis, renal failure, etc.) may be associated with epithelial ulceration, possible due to alteration of the mucus barrier.

Prognosis and treatment

Patients usually recover without any long-term complications. The removal of the offending cause is usually all that is required. An acute GI bleed should be treated in the conventional way. A proton pump inhibitor may be helpful in some cases.

PEPTIC ULCER DISEASE

Under this heading, we include gastritis, gastric ulcer and duodenal ulcer, which is dealt with here rather than in Chapter 16. These conditions are all associated with *H. pylori* infection.

Helicobacter pylori infection

Incidence

It is estimated that, in developed countries, 50% of the population over the age of 50 years are infected with the spiral-shaped Gram-negative bacterium. It appears that transmission occurs in childhood. The lower prevalence of *H. pylori* observed in younger people is a reflection of improved sanitation. In certain parts of the world (e.g. South America), the majority of the population is infected.

Clinical features

Asymptomatic infection is often discovered incidentally. Furthermore, the high prevalence of *H. pylori* infection in certain populations (e.g. Nigeria), without a concomitant, active disease process such as duodenal ulceration, indicates that host factors also have a role in producing pathology and symptoms.

Symptoms suggestive of acute gastritis, chronic gastritis or peptic ulcer disease usually unmask the presence of *H. pylori* (Fig. 15.3).

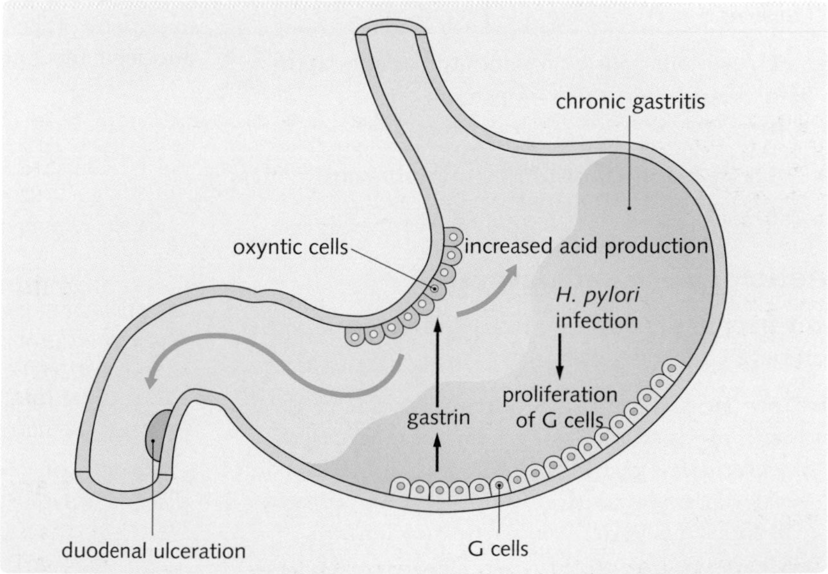

Fig. 15.3 Pathophysiological representation of mechanisms of *Helicobacter*-induced gastritis.

Epidemiological data suggest that there is an increased risk of gastric carcinoma, and long-standing gastritis increases the risk of gastric lymphoma.

Diagnosis and investigation

Non-invasive tests
Urea breath test:

- Most reliable test for diagnosis and confirming eradication after treatment.
- Urease from *H. pylori* acts on orally-administered ^{14}C or ^{13}C radiolabelled urea. Urea is broken down into ammonia and CO_2. The latter is detected in exhaled breath (see Fig. 24.8).

Serology:

- Immunoglobulin (Ig)G antibodies confirm past exposure rather than current infection.
- Not of value to confirm eradication.
- Stool antigen assay.

Invasive tests
These depend on endoscopy and biopsy and are highly sensitive and specific.
   Urease test:

- Antral biopsies are placed in a solution containing urea and a pH indicator. Urease activity produces ammonia which alters the pH. The subsequent colour change indicates a positive result.

Histology:

- *H. pylori* are visible on standard haematoxylin and eosin staining of biopsies.

Culture:

- May be helpful to confirm antibiotic sensitivities of *H. pylori*.

Aetiology and pathogenesis

The pattern of *H. pylori* infection influences its effect on peptic ulcer disease:

- Infection of the gastric antrum is associated with elevated levels of gastrin and increased secretion of gastric acid. There is an increased risk of duodenal ulcer in these patients due to increased acid delivery to the duodenum.

- Infection which involves the body of the stomach is associated with gastric ulceration, mucosal atrophy and reduced acid secretion. Body-predominant infection is associated with an increased risk of gastric cancer. Vitamin B_{12} deficiency may occur as a result of reduced intrinsic factor secretion due to atrophic gastritis.

Complications

- Acute GI bleed, due to peptic ulcer disease.
- Gastric lymphoma of a particular variety. 'Maltoma' has been associated with *Helicobacter* infection. This is a proliferative disease of the mucosa-associated lymphoid tissue (MALT). Reports of regression following *H. pylori* eradication therapy have been published.

Prognosis

Complete eradication is possible for most patients and reinfection rate is low.

Treatment

Different regimens have been described. The most successful regimens currently used involve triple therapy with two antibiotics and acid inhibition with a proton pump inhibitor. The antibiotics employed are a combination of amoxicillin, clarithromycin and metronidazole. Currently, this type of triple therapy regimen, employed as a twice-daily dose for 7 days, achieves eradication in approximately 90% of patients. (See text under treatment of gastric and duodenal ulceration.)

Any patient receiving metronidazole must avoid alcohol because the drug can inhibit acetaldehyde dehydrogenase and produce unpleasant histamine-induced symptoms if this metabolite builds up. This can manifest as facial flushing, headache, palpitations, vomiting and even cardiac arrhythmias.

Chronic gastritis

Incidence

- Can be a progression of acute gastritis.
- *H. pylori* gastritis is by far the most common aetiological factor.
- Autoimmune gastritis is associated with other autoimmune diseases.

Clinical features

- Most cases are asymptomatic.
- Symptoms are similar to those of acute gastritis, but occurring over a period of time.
- Pernicious anaemia due to loss of intrinsic factor secretion for vitamin B_{12} absorption occurs in patients with autoimmune gastritis.

Diagnosis and investigation

Endoscopy reveals an atrophic mucosa. Intrinsic factor autoantibodies and antiparietal cell antibodies are positive in patients with pernicious anaemia.

Aetiology and pathogenesis

- *H. pylori* is the commonest cause.
- NSAIDs.
- Alcohol.
- Autoimmune gastritis is an atrophic gastritis affecting mainly the body of the stomach. It is associated with antibodies to intrinsic factor and parietal cells. Pernicious anaemia may or may not be present.
- Bile reflux.

Complications

Intestinal metaplasia predisposes to malignancy.

Treatment

The aim is to treat the underlying cause:

- Eradication therapy for *H. pylori*.
- Stop NSAIDs and limit alcohol.

Gastric ulcer

Incidence

More commonly seen in the elderly population, gastric ulceration is less common than duodenal ulceration by a ratio of 1:4. Peak incidence occurs between 50 and 60 years of age.

Clinical features

Epigastric pain can be the main presenting feature. Classically, pain with gastric ulcer is associated with food, whereas duodenal ulcers tend to cause symptoms at night, or with an empty stomach, and are relieved by food. However, in the majority of cases, the discriminating value of these histories is poor and not helpful in the diagnosis.

Temporary relief with antacids is usually reported.

Associated features include nausea, heartburn, anorexia and weight loss. These symptoms also occur with gastric carcinoma.

Diagnosis and investigation

Investigations include:

- Endoscopy—the investigation of choice as biopsy enables differentiation of benign from malignant ulcers.
- Barium meal—will also demonstrate gastric and duodenal ulceration, but biopsies cannot be taken to exclude underlying malignancy.

Aetiology and pathogenesis

The exact aetiology is unknown, but *H. pylori* is present in 70% and most of the remainder are associated with NSAIDs. Some patients with gastric ulcers have normal or low acid output, especially ulcers occurring at the lesser curve. Theories regarding pathogenesis include:

- A possible defect in the mucosal barrier usually maintained by bicarbonate secretion by the gastric epithelium.
- Deficient prostaglandin-mediated cytoprotection. This may account for the higher incidence seen in elderly people because this cytoprotective mechanism diminishes with age.

Pre-pyloric ulcers are associated with a high acid output and behave more like a duodenal ulcer.

Differences between malignant and benign gastric ulcers are shown in Fig. 15.4.

Complications

- Iron-deficiency anaemia is common.
- Acute GI bleed, perforation or erosion can occur.
- Pre-pyloric ulcers may cause pyloric stenosis and resultant gastric outlet obstruction, but this is more commonly seen with duodenal ulcers.

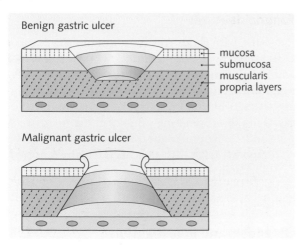

Benign gastric ulcer

mucosa
submucosa
muscularis
propria layers

Malignant gastric ulcer

Fig. 15.4 Differences between malignant and benign gastric ulcers. Usually benign ulcers are more superficial. Malignant ulcers have more heaped edges. Multiple biopsy is essential.

Iron-deficiency (hypochromic, microcytic) anaemia due to chronic blood loss is unusual in duodenal ulcers and, if present, coexisting pathology must be sought, such as carcinoma of the colon.

Prognosis

Fifty per cent of gastric ulcers recur within 1 year without *H. pylori* eradication.

Treatment

For *H. pylori* positive ulcers, a triple therapy eradication regimen, with acid suppression, is used. There is no known single best eradication regimen, but the following regimes are recommended by the British Society of Gastroenterology:

- One week duration: proton pump inhibitor (PPI) (standard dose twice daily), plus amoxicillin (1 g twice daily) or metronidazole (400 mg twice daily), plus clarithromycin (500 mg twice daily). It is sensible to avoid metronidazole if the patient has had a previous course of treatment with this agent.
- Second-line, quadruple therapy: PPI (standard dose twice daily), plus bismuth subcitrate (poorly tolerated), plus metronidazole (three times daily), plus tetracycline four times daily.

Compliance with treatment has been shown to be very important in determining the success of triple therapy regimens. The eradication course should be followed by antisecretory therapy for 2 months in gastric ulceration. Gastric ulcers tend to take longer to heal than duodenal ulcers.

Helicobacter pylori negative ulcers should be treated with standard antisecretory therapy for 2 months with cessation of NSAIDs where possible (see below).

Other strategies to aid healing include:

- Sulcralfate, which acts by mucosal protection against the action of pepsin; can be useful in resistant cases.
- Discourage smoking because it is linked to increased acid production.

Where NSAID use is clinically desirable, there are certain strategies that can be employed to reduce the risk of further mucosal damage:

- Use the lowest dose of NSAID required for symptom control.
- Misoprostol is a synthetic prostaglandin analogue with antisecretory and mucosal protective properties. It can help prevent NSAID-associated ulcers.
- Concomitant use of a PPI with NSAIDs is sometimes used in clinical practice, although this strategy is only recommended for those patients with a documented NSAID-induced ulcer who must unavoidably continue with NSAID therapy (e.g. severe rheumatoid arthritis) (as guided by the National Institute for Health and Clinical Excellence (NICE)).
- Cyclo-oxygenase 2 ('COX-2') selective inhibitors (e.g. celecoxib) have a significantly lower, but not zero, incidence of adverse upper GI effects. However, an increased risk of adverse cardiovascular side effects means that alternative analgesia should be sought in patients at risk of vascular disease.

Surgical treatment, such as partial gastrectomy and vagotomy, is reserved for complications of ulceration such as perforation or uncontrolled bleeding.

Dyspeptic symptoms are not a good indicator of the likelihood of a patient developing complications from taking NSAIDs. The majority of patients who have an ulcer or GI bleeding as a result of their NSAID have no warning symptoms prior to this.

Duodenal ulcer

Incidence

Approximately 15% of the population will have suffered from duodenal ulceration at some time.

Clinical features

- Epigastric pain (often intermittent).
- Classically, pain is said to be relieved by food or antacids and made worse by hunger.
- Patient can sometimes point to a specific site of pain in the epigastrium.
- May present as an acute GI bleed.

Diagnosis and investigation

As for gastric ulceration (i.e. endoscopy and biopsy, etc.). Tests for *H. pylori* infection should also be performed.

Aetiology and pathogenesis

Similar to that described for gastric ulceration (i.e. acid production, reduction in cytoprotection, etc.). The relationship between *H. pylori* infection and duodenal ulcers is more closely linked. Ninety-five per cent of patients with duodenal ulcers are infected with *H. pylori*. The exact pathogenic mechanism remains uncertain.

High acid output states are associated with duodenal ulceration as seen in Zollinger–Ellison syndrome. However, over two-thirds of patients have acid secretion within normal limits, which suggests that other factors, such as mucosal barrier and prostaglandin cytoprotection, are involved in its pathogenesis.

Environmental factors such as smoking and psychological stress are associated with increased basal output of acid, and NSAIDs reduce prostaglandin production, hence predisposing to ulceration.

First-degree relatives are at three times the normal risk of developing duodenal ulceration. Blood group O has a 40% increase in risk compared to the general population, especially those who do not secrete group O-related antigen in their gastric mucus glycoprotein.

Complications

Acute GI bleed, especially if there is an erosion of an artery. Perforation can present as an acute abdominal emergency and gastric outlet obstruction can occur with chronic disease.

Prognosis

Typically a recurrent disease, approximately 80% of patients relapse within 1 year if no maintenance or eradication therapy is given. Follow-up is not usually necessary in asymptomatic patients.

Treatment

The strategies taken are similar to those for gastric ulceration.

Confirmation of *H. pylori* infection is preferable before an eradication scheme is embarked upon. However, some authorities advocate eradication therapy should be given to all patients with duodenal ulceration because the correlation with *H. pylori* infection is so high.

NEOPLASIA OF THE STOMACH

Gastric polyps

Incidence

Adenomatous polyps are rare—discovered, often coincidentally, during approximately 2% of endoscopies.

Hyperplastic or cystic fundal polyps are common (85% of endoscopies).

Clinical features

The majority are asymptomatic. Occasionally, they may ulcerate and bleed.

Diagnosis and investigation

Investigations that may be of use include:

- Endoscopy for dyspepsia or abdominal pain—often identifies polyps incidentally. If multiple polyps are present, then conditions such as Peutz–Jeghers and familial polyposis coli should be considered. The latter has particular significance because of its malignant potential.
- Biopsy for histological examination—will usually confirm the nature of the polyp.
- Endoscopic ultrasound—may be necessary to exclude submucosal malignant infiltration.

Aetiology and pathogenesis

- Hyperplastic polyps are non-sinister.

- Approximately 5% of polyps are adenomas and have similar pre-malignant potential as those found in the colon.

Rarely, patients with pernicious anaemia have polyps in the fundus, which subsequently turn out to be carcinoid tumours. These may be due to the trophic effects of gastrin secondary to achlorhydria.

Complications

Bleeding and malignant change are the usual complications.

Prognosis and treatment

Resection of the polyp will abolish the malignant risk. They can be removed endoscopically via a snare, but those that are large or sessile may not be suitable, hence multiple biopsies are usually taken and local surgical resection may be required. Hyperplastic polyps are usually left alone unless the patient is symptomatic (Fig. 15.5).

Gastrointestinal stromal tumours

Gastrointestinal stromal tumours (GISTs) account for 80% of gastrointestinal mesenchymal tumours. Before 2000, GISTs were variably classified as leiomyomas, leiomyosarcomas, leiomyoblastomas, Schwannomas or gastrointestinal autonomic nerve tumours. Gastrointestinal stromal tumours are within the wall of the stomach (intramural) but arise below the mucosa (submucosal) so overlying mucosa can be intact.

Incidence

Gastrointestinal stromal tumours are rare, accounting for 3% of GI tract malignancies. Fifty to seventy per cent occur in the stomach.

Clinical features

- Asymptomatic if small.
- GI blood loss if they ulcerate and bleed.
- Abdominal pain.
- Palpable mass.

Diagnosis and investigation

- Endoscopy—50% have an intragastric component and are visible at endoscopy. It may appear as a submucosal tumour covered by intact mucosa or have an ulcerated surface.

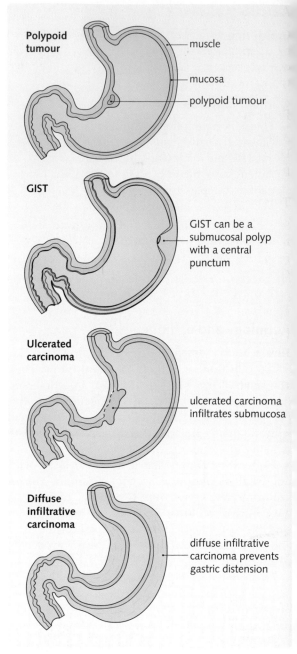

Fig. 15.5 Types of gastric polyps and contrast with GI stromal tumour (GIST) and carcinoma.

- Endoscopic ultrasound (EUS)—helps characterize submucosal masses and EUS-guided fine needle aspiration may allow diagnosis.
- CT scanning—useful to evaluate size and assess for evidence of spread.

Aetiology and pathogenesis

Gastrointestinal stromal tumours are characterized by mutations in the c-kit proto-oncogene causing overactivity of a membrane receptor-associated tyrosine kinase.

Prognosis

All GISTs are considered to be potentially malignant. Larger size is associated with increased malignant potential.

Treatment

Surgical resection may be curative. Imatinib (an oral monoclonal antibody against the tyrosine kinase receptor) is used to treat non-resectable malignant GISTs.

Ménétrièr's disease

Incidence

Rare.

Clinical features

These include:

- Abdominal pain, vomiting or bleeding similar to those of chronic gastritis.
- Hypoalbuminaemia due to protein loss from the gastric mucosa.

Diagnosis and investigation

Endoscopy demonstrates the typical appearance of enlarged, thickened folds of mucosa.

Aetiology and pathogenesis

Unknown aetiology—normal gastric mucosa is replaced by hypertrophied epithelium producing a characteristic appearance. It is not a true 'neoplasia', but can be very difficult to differentiate macroscopically from infiltrating neoplasms.

Histologically, there is hyperplasia of the mucin-producing glands with glandular proliferation, together with loss of parietal and chief cells (Fig. 15.6). Excessive protein loss occurs through the gastric mucosa as a consequence of mucus secretion.

Complications

The condition is possibly pre-malignant but the risk is poorly characterized.

Treatment

Treatment includes:

- Antisecretory medication—may be of help to some patients.
- Partial gastrectomy—may be required to reduce the amount of protein loss.

Gastric carcinoma

Incidence

The frequency of gastric carcinoma increases with age and affects approximately 15 out of 100 000 people in the UK. There is a higher incidence in Japan and the Far East for which dietary factors have been implicated.

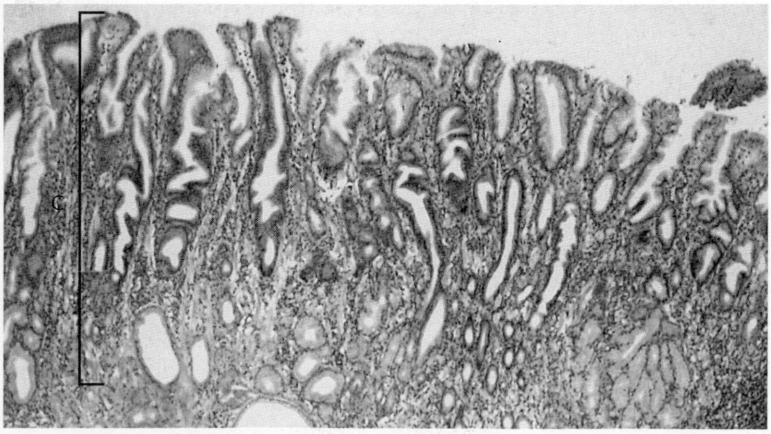

Fig. 15.6 Ménétrièr's disease. The gastric mucosa is grossly thickened due to hypertrophy. Note elongated crypts (C).

Clinical features

These include:

- Abdominal pain with a nature similar to that of peptic ulceration, but progressive and severe, if local invasion has occurred.
- Weight loss—often profound and may be the only presenting complaint.
- Nausea, vomiting and anorexia—these are common features. If the tumour is close to the pylorus, then vomiting can be marked due to gastric outlet obstruction.
- Anaemia—this can be iron deficient as a result of occult blood loss, reflect chronic disease or rarely bone marrow infiltration with metastases.
- Distant metastases (e.g. to brain, bone, liver and lung) produce symptoms and variable clinical presentations according to site.

Up to 50% of patients will have a palpable epigastric mass at presentation. Supraclavicular lymph nodes behind the left sternomastoid muscle (Virchow's node) can be palpated in one-third of patients. Other physical signs (all suggestive of incurable disease) include hepatomegaly, jaundice, ascites and paraneoplastic skin manifestations such as acanthosis nigricans.

Diagnosis and investigation

Relevant investigations include:

- Endoscopy—this is the investigation of choice. All gastric ulcers should be biopsied to exclude malignancy. Repeat endoscopy a few weeks later should be performed to confirm healing. A non-healing ulcer raises the possibility of malignancy.
- Barium meal—in the investigation of dyspepsia, a barium meal may show a gastric ulcer, or a diffuse infiltrative type of gastric cancer may be seen as a rigid, contracted stomach.
- Computed tomography (CT) scan is undertaken in proven or suspected cases to look for evidence of local or metastatic spread.
- Positron emission tomography (PET) scan is also being used to assess for spread.
- Biochemical tests may demonstrate derangement of liver enzymes, if liver metastases are present, or hypercalcaemia suggesting bony metastasis.

Aetiology and pathogenesis

- Chronic *H. pylori* infection is associated with an increased risk of gastric cancer. It causes gastric atrophy which is associated with a 2.5-fold increase in risk of gastric cancer.
- Diet—at neutral pH, nitrites are converted to nitrosamines which are known to be carcinogenic in animals. The high incidence of gastric cancer in China and Japan appears to be diet related. (The incidence is lower in migrants from these countries.)
- Pernicious anaemia has an increased risk of gastric cancer, possibly due to achlorhydria.
- Blood group A carries a 20% increased risk of gastric cancer.
- Previous partial gastrectomy carries an increased risk of gastric cancer after 20 years.
- Lower socioeconomic classes have a higher incidence. *H. pylori* infection may be a confounding factor.
- Adenomatous gastric polyps are rare, but they are pre-malignant and should be removed.

Two histological types of gastric cancer have been described:

- Glandular adenocarcinoma, similar to that seen throughout the intestine with well-differentiated glandular formation or acini which secrete mucin.
- Diffuse, spreading-type adenocarcinoma with a fibrous stroma giving a fibrotic appearance to the stomach (linitis plastica or 'leather-bottle' stomach).

Prognosis

Carcinomas that are confined to the mucosa (rare) have a 90% 5-year survival compared with invasive lesions, which have less than 10% 5-year survival. Early detection appears to be possible in screening programmes such as those in Japan, where gastric carcinoma is common.

Treatment

Ideally, cases are discussed by a multidisciplinary team that includes a pathologist, surgeon, radiologist, gastroenterologist, oncologist, specialist nurse and other allied health professionals.

Options for treatment include:

- Surgery—this is the only treatment that can offer a cure. This ranges from partial gastrectomy to radical resection with local lymph node clearance, but is only suitable for patients without widespread metastases. Palliative procedures to relieve outlet obstruction may be appropriate.

- Chemotherapy and radiotherapy—these are not usually of use but may be helpful for control of symptoms due to tumour bulk.
- Symptom control with opiate analgesia and antiemetics—can be difficult to achieve.

Gastric lymphoma

Incidence

Accounts for 5–10% of all gastric malignancy in the UK.

Clinical features

Similar to those of gastric carcinoma. Drenching night sweats may also be a prominent feature.

Diagnosis and investigation

Endoscopy and biopsy will provide a histological diagnosis. CT of the thorax, abdomen and pelvis looks for extra-GI lymphadenopathy and splenomegaly. Bone marrow biopsy, particularly indicated if full blood count (FBC) is abnormal, provides evidence of marrow involvement with lymphoma. Serum lactate dehydrogenase may be elevated.

Aetiology and pathogenesis

Nearly all are of non-Hodgkin's B cell type arising from mucosal-associated lymphoid tissue (MALT), rather than a primary lymph node tumour. These tumours are associated with *H. pylori*.

Prognosis

Very good, with 80–90% survival depending on the type of lymphoma. Complete excision of the tumour can be curative.

Treatment

Treatment options include:

- Eradication therapy for *H. pylori*, which can produce regression of certain types.
- Chemotherapy and radiotherapy, which may be necessary for aggressive 'high-grade' transformation or relapsed disease.
- Surgical resection of the tumour.

- Endoscopic surveillance to monitor response to treatment or for interval biopsies is undertaken by some clinicians.

Gastroparesis

Clinical features

Vomiting and nausea are the main symptoms. Weight loss may ensue if the patient avoids eating.

Diagnosis and investigation

Investigations include:

- Barium meal—demonstrates distension of the stomach with markedly reduced passage of barium into the duodenum.
- Radioisotope scan—this is an alternative to a barium meal.

Aetiology and pathogenesis

Characterized by reduced motility of the stomach. Causes include previous surgical vagotomy (now rarely performed) or autonomic neuropathy complicating diabetes mellitus. In some cases, no identifiable cause is found.

Complications

Those associated with prolonged vomiting (hypokalaemia, aspiration pneumonia) and malnutrition.

Treatment

- Antiemetics with a prokinetic action such as domperidone or metoclopramide are often used to enhance gastric emptying. In severe cases, a motilin analogue such as erythromycin may be required. Clearly, the underlying cause should be addressed where possible.
- Gastic pacemaker—electrical stimulation to induce gastric motility is being used in selected patients with refractory symptoms.

Gastric outlet obstruction

Incidence

Affects up to 3% of patients with duodenal or pre-pyloric ulceration.

Crohn's disease

Crohn's disease is a form of inflammatory bowel disease that can involve any location of the alimentary tract from the mouth to the anus. The inflammation of Crohn's disease is often discontinuous with normal sections of gut between inflamed areas ('skip lesions'). Inflammation may affect all layers of the gut from the mucosa to the serosa.

Crohn's disease most commonly affects the terminal ileum and proximal large bowel (Fig. 16.3).

Incidence and prevalence

- Incidence: 5–10 per 100 000 per year.
- Prevalence: 50–100 per 100 000.

There is a peak incidence of Crohn's disease at 15–30 years, with a median age of diagnosis of 30 years.

Clinical features

The clinical features of Crohn's disease are varied and depend on the site of disease, activity of disease and disease behaviour.

General points

- Constitutional symptoms (malaise, weight loss and fever) may reflect severe disease. These are occasionally the sole presenting symptoms in Crohn's disease.

- Pain is more frequent and a more persistent complaint than in ulcerative colitis.
- Rectal bleeding—gross rectal bleeding is uncommon.
- Weight loss due to malabsorption (ileal resection or dysfunction) or poor oral intake, for example.
- Systemic manifestations (Fig. 16.4).
- A 'cobblestone' appearance of the mucosa can occur in Crohn's disease as a consequence of deep ulceration and fissuring.
- Diarrhoea.

Multiple factors may contribute to diarrhoea in Crohn's disease:

- Bile salt-induced diarrhoea/steatorrhoea (due to ileal resection or dysfunction).
- Bacterial overgrowth.
- Disordered colonic motility secondary to chronic inflammation.
- Altered fluid and electrolyte absorption and secretion.
- Exudation of protein and fluid from mucosal wall.

Clinical features according to location of disease

- Ileal disease (often with accompanying caecal involvement).
- Small bowel obstruction.
- Fibrotic stricture—colicky, intermittent abdominal pain and/or nausea and vomiting.

Fig. 16.3 Gastrointestinal features of Crohn's disease.

mouth of oesophageal ulcers are common

gastroduodenal 1–2%

transmural inflammation with non-caseating granulomas

skip lesions with normal areas in between are characteristic

small bowel alone 30%

ileocolonic or entero-enteral anastomoses are common

ileocolonic 40–50%

colon alone 20–30%

the rectum is usually spared

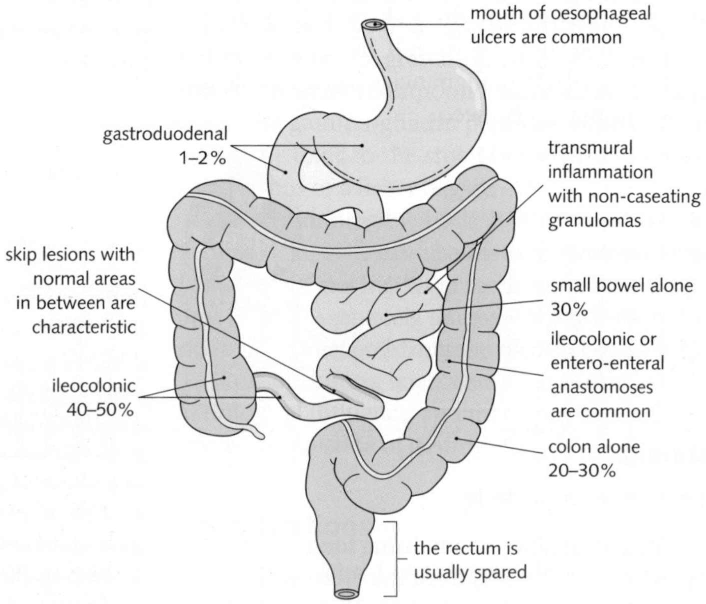

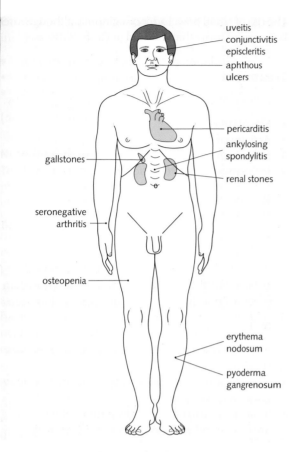

Fig. 16.4 Systemic manifestations of Crohn's disease.

- Fullness/mass in right iliac fossa.
- Loose stool.

Colonic disease and perianal disease (see Ch. 17):

- Stool may be bloody depending on extent/severity of disease.

Upper gastrointestinal tract lesions (uncommon in absence of disease beyond the duodeno-jejunal junction):

- Gastroduodenal—dyspepsia, epigastric pain; outflow obstruction (oedema/fibrotic stricture) with early satiety, nausea and vomiting.
- Oesophageal (<2%)—dysphagia, odynophagia, chest pain, heartburn.
- Jejunum and ileum—frank malabsorption and steatorrhoea.

Clinical features according to behaviour of disease
- Stricturing disease—may be asymptomatic until the luminal calibre is small enough to cause relative obstruction.

- Penetrating disease—fistulating Crohn's disease (perianal fistulae; communicating fistulae between intestine and other organs or abdominal wall).
- Abscess formation—may affect 25% of Crohn's patients at some point. Patients may have spiking temperatures and focal abdominal tenderness.

Diagnosis and investigation

The role of investigations in Crohn's disease is to:

1. Establish the diagnosis.
2. Establish the extent of disease.
3. Establish the site and extent of stricturing disease.
4. Establish the activity of disease.
5. Detect extramural complications (e.g. abscesses and fistulae).

The history and examination will guide the choice of test.

Blood tests in Crohn's disease
- C-reactive protein—broadly correlates with disease activity.
- Haemoglobin—a number of factors may contribute towards anaemia in Crohn's disease, for example malabsorption (vitamin B_{12} and folate deficiency), bleeding and azathioprine.

C-reactive protein is elevated during acute attacks, mirroring inflammatory activity in Crohn's disease, and is useful for monitoring response to treatment.

Endoscopic investigations
Endoscopic investigations allow biopsy to aid diagnosis:

- Colonoscopy—allows intubation of the terminal ileum.
- Gastroscopy—if upper GI symptoms.
- Wireless capsule enteroscopy (see Ch. 24)—does not allow biopsy but produces images of bowel that are beyond the reach of conventional endoscopy.

Fig. 17.1 Anatomy of the large intestine.

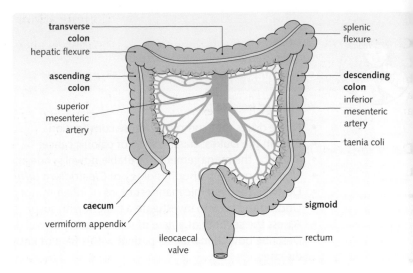

count, biochemistry and inflammatory markers will be normal.

Further investigations are necessary if there is a suspicion of an underlying pathology.

Indicators that other diseases should be excluded before diagnosing IBS include:

- A short history of symptoms.
- Weight loss.
- Nocturnal symptoms.
- Rectal bleeding.
- Age over 50 years.

Aetiology and pathogenesis

Factors that have been implicated in the mechanism of IBS include:

- Abnormal gastrointestinal (GI) sensation.
- Abnormal GI motility.
- Altered GI serotonin signalling.
- Altered bacterial flora.

Complications

There is no evidence that IBS leads to more serious GI diseases.

Treatment

Patients with IBS require reassurance, explanation and lifestyle advice.

Reassurance and tactful explanation are pivotal to the management of these patients, and it must be

emphasized that the disorder does not progress to a more serious disease.

Treatment options include:

- Treatment of anxiety and depression. Tricyclic antidepressants may help pain at doses lower than those used to treat depression.
- Antispasmodics, e.g. mebeverine.
- Peppermint oil—can help bloating.
- Increased fibre and fluid intake in constipation-predominant IBS.
- A trial of excluding certain foods (e.g. dairy, wheat, etc.) —can be helpful, but is difficult to implement and should be done so under the supervision of a dietician.
- Hypnotherapy—can have lasting benefit (but is not widely available).

Opioids should be avoided as they may make symptoms worse.

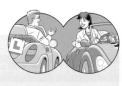

A diagnosis of IBS can often be made at the first consultation. The diagnosis of IBS should be given in a positive way, rather than as a diagnosis of exclusion. More than 50% of IBS patients believe they have serious disease and these concerns should be carefully explored with the patient, preferably at an early consultation.

Megacolon

Clinical features

Constipation is characteristic, with a long, protracted history possibly with faecal impaction and soiling at a young age. Reduced rectal sensation is usual and anal tone may be increased on rectal examination.

Diagnosis and investigation

Investigations to consider:

- Barium enema or plain abdominal X-ray shows a dilated proximal colon. A narrowed distal colon may be seen in Hirschsprung's disease.
- Deep mucosal rectal biopsy is necessary, especially in young patients, to confirm or exclude Hirschsprung's disease in which a segment of the rectum has absent or reduced ganglion cells in the submucosa.
- Manometry shows failure of internal sphincter relaxation in response to rectal distension.

Aetiology and pathogenesis

The condition can be congenital or acquired.

Congenital type is known as Hirschsprung's disease, which usually presents in childhood with chronic constipation and faecal soiling. Rectal biopsy shows an absence of ganglion cells in the submucosal plexus. Adults presenting with the condition may have segmental disease, hence initial biopsy may be normal and a deeper biopsy or a full-thickness biopsy is required.

The most common cause of acquired megacolon is chronic constipation with or without laxative abuse. Causes of chronic constipation are many (Fig. 17.2). Chronic ingestion of laxatives results in depletion of ganglion cells.

Fig. 17.2 Causes of chronic constipation

Low residue diet
Drugs, e.g. opioids, iron, anti-depressants
Metabolic conditions: hypothyroidism, hypercalcaemia
Neuropsychiatric conditions: Parkinson's, depression, stroke (immobility)
Obstruction and pseudo-obstruction
Painful anorectal conditions, e.g. fissure
Carcinoma of the colon

Complications

Subacute or acute bowel obstruction can ensue.

Treatment

Hirschsprung's disease is primarily treated by surgical resection of the affected colon.

Acquired megacolon is more difficult to treat because patients may have been taking laxatives for some time. Frequent enemas or manual evacuations may be needed. In severe cases, surgical intervention is required.

Pseudo-obstruction

Clinical features

Similar to those of bowel obstruction (i.e. vomiting, distension, non-passage of flatus, etc.), but unlike true obstruction, bowel sounds are absent.

Aetiology and pathogenesis

Bowel paralysis is common after laparotomy due to manual handling and will return to normal within 2–3 days. Systemic conditions can also give rise to an adynamic bowel (e.g. drugs, electrolyte disturbance, septicaemia). It is commonly seen in intensive care patients.

Treatment

Correction of the underlying abnormality will usually result in the return of normal peristalsis.

INFLAMMATORY BOWEL DISEASE

Crohn's disease and ulcerative colitis are inflammatory conditions of the bowel characterized by periods of remission and relapse. Both conditions appear to be an inflammatory response to environmental triggers in genetically susceptible individuals.

Ulcerative colitis is confined to the colon, whereas Crohn's disease may affect any part of the GI tract from the mouth to the anus. They have overlapping features and share some treatment strategies. In some patients, it can be difficult to distinguish colonic Crohn's disease from ulcerative colitis.

Ulcerative colitis

Ulcerative colitis is a form of inflammatory bowel disease which is limited to the colon. It affects the

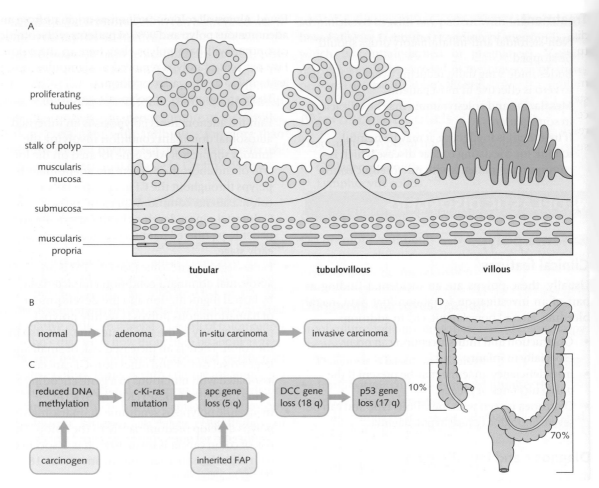

Fig. 17.9 (A) Types of colonic polyps. (B) A summary of the polyp cancer sequence in the colon. (C) Molecular changes involved. (D) Two-thirds of colon cancers occur within 60 cm of the anal verge and within reach of a flexible sigmoidoscope. (FAP, familial adenomatous polyposis.)

ideally be removed to prevent malignant transformation (see Fig. 24.18).
- Surgical resection if individual polyps cannot be removed.
- Surveillance of patients who are at risk (i.e. polyposis coli and their first-degree relatives).
- Colonoscopic screening for those who have had a colonic adenoma—undertaken according to size and number of polyps (assigned low, intermediate or high risk). For example, one or two adenomas measuring

<1 cm may only need one screen after 5 years, whereas multiple large polyps require annual colonoscopy.

Colorectal carcinoma

Incidence

The second most common carcinoma in the UK affects approximately 20 out of 100 000 people. Mean age at diagnosis is between 60 and 65 years. Disease is rare in Africa and Asia and this is thought to be linked to environmental rather than genetic factors.

Aetiology and pathogenesis

Western diets of high animal fat and low fibre have been linked to colorectal carcinoma, possibly due to slow transit of intestinal content which increases contact time between potential carcinogens and the bowel wall.

Always be alerted by a history of sustained change in bowel habit, particularly in those over 45 years. Colonic carcinoma should be excluded in this setting.

Familial polyposis coli and inflammatory bowel disease are risk factors for the development of colonic tumours.

Colonic carcinoma is thought to be a result of multiple genetic alterations that occur in a progressive, stepwise manner. Oncogenes that normally regulate cell division and differentiation undergo mutation as a result of external stimuli. Mutation of the APC tumour-suppressor gene on the long arm of chromosome 5 seems to promote the development of adenomas. This is the inherited defect in familial adenomatous polyposis. The progression from adenoma to carcinoma involves mutations in other oncogenes, e.g. K-*ras*, p53, etc. (see Fig. 17.9). Dukes' classification of colonic cancer is shown in Figure 17.10.

Lesions occurring in the descending colon tend to be annular and produce the typical 'apple-core' lesion on barium enema (see Fig. 24.25).

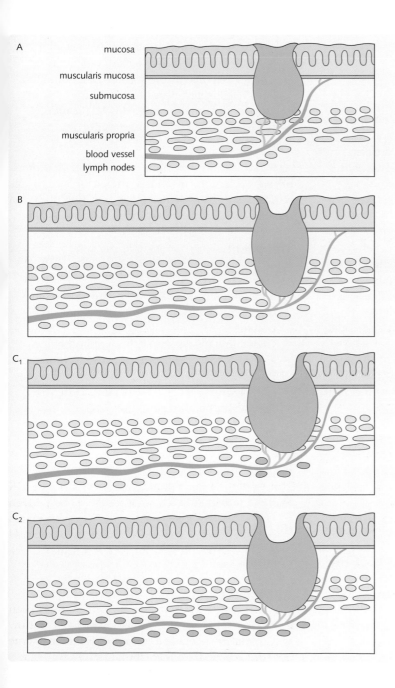

Fig. 17.10 Dukes' classification of colonic cancer. (A) The tumour is confined to the bowel wall; (B) it extends through the muscle coat but does not involve lymph nodes; (C) all layers are affected, with the proximal lymph node affected in C_1 and both the proximal and the highest resected nodes positive in C_2.

A
mucosa
muscularis mucosa
submucosa
muscularis propria
blood vessel
lymph nodes

B

C_1

C_2

The tumours produce a variable amount of mucin and, histologically, signet ring cells can be seen where the nucleus is pushed to one side due to cytoplasmic mucus.

Hereditary non-polyposis colorectal cancer (HNPCC) is an autosomal dominant disorder in which colon cancer develops from flat adenomas (i.e. without polyp formation). The underlying genetic defect is in one of the DNA mismatch repair (MMR) genes, e.g. hMSH2, hMLH1.

- It accounts for 6% of colon cancers.
- Cancers are mainly right-sided.
- The peak incidence of cancer is 40 years.
- Most cases are due to mutations in genes responsible for repair of errors in DNA replications (mismatch repair genes).
- HNPCC in which cancers are limited to the colon is called Lynch syndrome type I.
- HNPCC in which family members are also prone to cancers of the female genital tract and other sites is called Lynch syndrome type II.

Clinical features

The main features are:

- Anaemia, weight loss, abdominal pain, or loose bowel motions—the most common features. A mass may be palpable in the right iliac fossa, especially with caecal lesions. Rectal bleeding or obstruction is more common with left-sided lesions (e.g. rectosigmoid).
- Altered bowel habit—seen in >50% of all patients.
- Perforation and abscess formation—not uncommon, and jaundice due to liver metastases can occur in advanced cases.

Rectal examination is a mandatory part of the examination as a tumour can often be palpated.

Diagnosis and investigation

Investigations of use include:

- Full blood count—may detect iron-deficiency anaemia, which is common.
- Faecal occult blood—is often positive but can be seen in any cause of underlying GI bleed (e.g. duodenal ulceration). It is used as part of the screening test for bowel cancer.
- Barium enema—is still the investigation of choice in most centres because of its wide availability.

- Rigid sigmoidoscopy—only identifies rectosigmoid tumours.
- Flexible sigmoidoscopy—can detect up to 70% of tumours and is a better investigation in combination with barium enema to examine the remainder of the colon.
- Colonoscopy allows direct inspection of colonic mucosa and allows biopsy of mucosal lesions.
- Abdominal ultrasound—is sensitive for detecting metastases in the liver before surgical resection.
- Computed tomography (CT) colonography—uses contrast medium in the colonic lumen to outline mucosal abnormalities. It is useful if a patient's poor mobility precludes their having a barium enema or colonoscopy. It requires full bowel cleansing before the procedure.
- Magnetic resonance imaging (MRI) scanning—can be helpful to assess resectability of rectal tumours.

A bowel cancer screening programme has been developed in the UK and is offered in specific age bands. Screened patients have a faecal occult blood test, and those that test positive undergo colonoscopy.

Treatment

The mainstays of management are:

- Surgical resection with end-to-end anastomosis or end colostomy, depending on the site of the tumour.
- Chemotherapy with or without radiotherapy—given to patients with Dukes' B and C, which can improve survival (see Fig. 17.10). Chemotherapy can sometimes be given to patients with liver metastases, but the results are disappointing.

Prognosis

See Figure 17.11. Overall survival is 30% at 5 years.

Angiodysplasia

Incidence

Relatively rare condition affecting the elderly population.

Clinical features

To note:

- Chronic iron-deficiency anaemia is due to chronic blood loss from the GI tract.

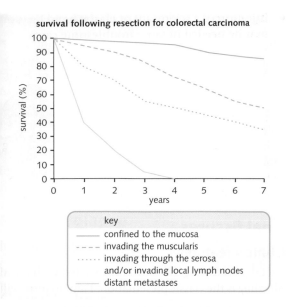

survival following resection for colorectal carcinoma

key
— confined to the mucosa
- - - invading the muscularis
...... invading through the serosa
and/or invading local lymph nodes
— distant metastases

Fig. 17.11 Survival following resection for colorectal carcinoma according to Dukes' staging. Note that survival is commensurate with that of the normal population if the tumour is confined to the mucosa.

- Acute GI bleeding can occur, causing hypotension and shock in some patients.

Diagnosis and investigation

Diagnosis can be difficult and often involves repeated gastroscopy and colonoscopy to detect the lesion:

- Red cell radioisotope-labelled scanning can be helpful to identify the site of blood loss.
- Selective angiography may demonstrate abnormal blood vessels or the site of active bleeding if the blood loss is >0.5 mL/min.

Aetiology and pathogenesis

The underlying aetiology is unknown but the condition is most likely to be acquired because it affects mainly the elderly population. There is an association with aortic stenosis (Heyde's syndrome), and approximately half the patients will have some form of cardiac disease. It can exist anywhere along the GI tract, but is more commonly found in the proximal colon, caecum and terminal ileum.

Treatment

Electrocoagulation or argon photocoagulation during colonoscopy can be successful for small lesions. Larger proximal lesions will need surgical resection. Hormonal treatment with oestrogen derivatives can result in regression of the lesions. The anti-angiogenic drug, thalidomide, has also been shown to be effective in some patients.

ANORECTAL CONDITIONS

Haemorrhoids

Clinical features

The main symptoms are:

- Rectal bleeding, which may coat the stools or drip into the toilet at the end of defecation.
- Perianal irritation and itching.

Diagnosis and investigation

Proctoscopy reveals haemorrhoids, classically at the 3, 7 and 11 o'clock positions with the patient supine in a trendelenberg position.

Aetiology and pathogenesis

Haemorrhoids result from enlargement of the venous plexuses at the lower end of the anal mucosa.

Raised intra-abdominal pressure inhibits venous return to the vena cava and hence causes venous engorgement. Common contributing factors are constipation, pregnancy, excessive straining to pass urine or stool, etc.

A minor degree of rectal prolapse is common. Oestrogen-related venous dilatation may also contribute to development of haemorrhoids in pregnancy.

Rectal bleeding occurs as a result of trauma by passage of hard stools. Symptoms are usually intermittent and exacerbated by constipation.

Mucus secreted by glandular epithelium can block skin pores, which causes secondary infection by bacteria and *Candida*, followed by local skin irritation. Haemorrhoids are classified as first, second and third degree, as shown in Figure 17.12. They may be painful if they thrombose.

Complications

Thrombosis of the haemorrhoids is painful and irreducible. However, it is a self-limiting condition that eventually results in atrophy and fibrosis of the thrombosed haemorrhoids, leaving visible anal tags.

- Antibiotic use.
- Old age.
- Comorbidity.

Treatment

Oral metronidazole is usually used as first-line treatment. Vancomycin is also effective and is often used for recurrent infection.

Prognosis

Mortality of up to 30% has been described in hospitalized patients with *C. difficile*.

Amoebiasis

Incidence

Occurs worldwide, but more commonly in the tropics.

Clinical features

In acute infection, these include:

- Abdominal pain.
- Diarrhoea (often bloody).
- Nausea and vomiting.

Fulminant colitis and toxic dilatation rarely can occur.

Diagnosis and investigation

Investigations:

- Fresh stool samples are required for identification of amoebic cysts.
- Specific antibody can be measured in the serum.
- Sigmoidoscopy demonstrates ulceration of the colonic mucosa but it is not diagnostic.

Aetiology and pathogenesis

The disease is caused by *Entamoeba histolytica* which is digested in its cyst form via contaminated food or water, or direct person-to-person spread. Multiplication of the organism takes place in the colon, where they invade the colonic epithelium, causing ulceration. Not all who are infected will have clinical disease, and some become asymptomatic cyst carriers.

Complications

Uncommon—perforation due to toxic dilatation can occur. Strictures can occur in chronic infection.

Hepatic abscesses are not uncommon (see Ch. 18).

Treatment

Metronidazole is the drug of choice. Education and advice regarding hygiene can help reduce person-to-person spread.

Cryptosporidiosis

Clinical features

Symptoms include:

- Watery diarrhoea.
- Fever.
- Abdominal pain.

Toxic dilatation and sclerosing cholangitis can be seen in patients with AIDS.

Diagnosis and investigation

Parasite can be identified by modified Ziehl–Nielsen stain of faeces or intestinal biopsy. Faecal oocysts should be quantified.

Aetiology and pathogenesis

The fungal parasite is found worldwide with its major reservoir in cattle, and is likely to be spread via contaminated water supplies.

Healthy individuals will have a self-limiting gastro-enteritis and often the diagnosis is not confirmed. People who are immunocompromised tend to have a devastating illness with protracted episodes of diarrhoea.

The organism also causes sclerosing cholangitis in the immunocompromised patient.

Treatment

It may be self-limiting if the CD4 lymphocyte count is not too suppressed. Paromomycin has been shown to be effective. Good hygiene prevents spread of the infection.

Schistosomiasis

See also Chapter 18 and Figure 18.28.

Clinical features

The main features are:

- Fever.
- Urticaria.
- Nausea.
- Vomiting.
- Bloody diarrhoea.

Diagnosis and investigation

Consider the following investigations:

- Specific antibodies can be detected by serology.
- Eggs can be isolated from stool, urine or rectal biopsy.
- Sigmoidoscopy reveals mucosal ulceration which, as an isolated finding, is not diagnostic.

Aetiology and pathogenesis

Schistosoma mansoni predominantly affects the colon, causing erythema and ulceration of the mucosa. A localized granulomatous reaction may be mistaken for colonic cancer. Progressive fibrosis leads to stricture formation but obstruction is rare.

Schistosoma japonicum affects the small intestine and proximal colon, and epithelial dysplasia is seen with chronic infection which is now accepted to be a premalignant condition.

Complications

- Peri-portal fibrosis and portal hypertension can ensue.
- Ectopic deposition of eggs elsewhere in the body (e.g. lung and brain).

Treatment

The drug of choice is praziquantel, as it is effective against all human schistosomes, combining broad-spectrum activity with low toxicity.

Whipworm infection

Incidence

Found worldwide and the prevalence can be as high as 90% in poor communities with poor hygiene.

Clinical features

Usually asymptomatic.

Heavy infestation causes bloody diarrhoea associated with weight loss, abdominal discomfort and anorexia. Involvement of the appendix causes appendicitis.

Diagnosis and investigation

- Stool examination for eggs.
- Sigmoidoscopy—adult worms may be seen attached to the rectal mucosa.

Aetiology and pathogenesis

Caused by *Trichuris trichura*. Adult worms are more commonly found in the distal ileum and caecum. The whole colon may be affected in heavy infection.

The adult worm embeds itself in the colonic mucosa, causing damage and ulceration, leading to protein and blood loss in severe cases.

Treatment

The anthelmintic mebendazole is the treatment of choice, but its use needs to be combined with hygienic measures to break the cycle of auto-infection. All family members should receive therapy.

Threadworm infection

Incidence

Occurs worldwide, but is more prevalent in temperate climates. Outbreaks are seen in institutional establishments and areas of overcrowded living conditions.

Clinical features

- Pruritus ani is intense and usually nocturnal due to egg laying by the female worm.
- Submucosal abscess is rare and due to secondary bacterial infection of the colonic mucosa.

Diagnosis and investigation

Adult worms may be seen directly leaving the anus. Clear adhesive tape can be applied to the peri-anal region to allow the identification of eggs microscopically.

Aetiology and pathogenesis

Caused by *Enterobius vermicularis* and commonly affects children. Adult worms reside in the colon and female worms migrate to the peri-anal region to lay their eggs. Superficial damage to the colonic mucosa is common during heavy infestations.

Autoinfection via scratching and poor hygiene aggravates the problem. Rarely, migration to the peritoneum and visceral organs occurs.

be distinguished from Dubin–Johnson syndrome by a normal liver biopsy. Prognosis is also excellent for this syndrome.

VIRAL HEPATITIS

Traditionally, viruses with a predilection to cause hepatitis have come to be classified alphabetically. Currently, at least six different viruses are known to infect humans (A, B, C, D, E and G). Other viruses such as cytomegalovirus (CMV), Epstein–Barr virus (EBV), yellow fever and herpes viruses can also infect the liver.

Hepatitis A

Incidence

This is the most common type of hepatitis worldwide, with the young most frequently afflicted. Epidemics are associated with overcrowding, poor hygiene and sanitation. Transmission is by the faecal–oral route or ingestion of contaminated water or shellfish.

Clinical features

In the prodromal phase:

- Symptoms mimic viral gastroenteritis (nausea, vomiting, diarrhoea, headache, mild fever, malaise and abdominal discomfort).
- There is a distaste for cigarettes said to be characteristic in young adults who normally smoke them.

The icteric phase occurs after 10–14 days (some patients remain anicteric) and resolves in 2–3 weeks:

- Mild symptoms such as malaise and fatigue may persist for months.
- Liver enlargement is common during the icteric phase; the spleen is palpable in approximately 10%.

Diagnosis and investigation

Diagnosis is usually made on clinical grounds. A definitive diagnosis can be made if there is a rising titre of anti-hepatitis A virus (anti-HAV) immunoglobulin (Ig)M and/or demonstration of viral particles in stools by electron microscopy. Elevated anti-HAV IgG titre reflects previous exposure to hepatitis A and thus lifelong immunity. Transaminases are moderately elevated (500–1000 IU/L) but normalize rapidly (Fig. 18.3).

Aetiology and pathogenesis

Hepatitis A is a pico-RNA-virus excreted in the faeces of an infected person approximately 2 weeks before the onset of jaundice and up to 1 week thereafter. The disease is most infectious just prior to the onset of jaundice. The RNA virus is relatively heat resistant withstanding 60°C for up to 30 minutes, hence it thrives in areas of poor hygiene.

Complications

Rare, but myocarditis, arthritis, vasculitis and, very occasionally, fulminant hepatic failure have been described.

Prognosis

Most patients recover completely without any sequelae; some have a self-limiting relapse of

Fig. 18.3 Laboratory tests and their time course in hepatitis A infection.

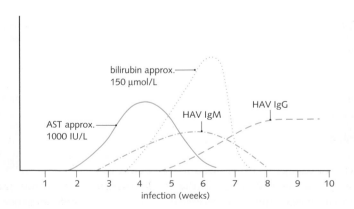

hepatitis. A few have a prolonged cholestatic jaundice (3–4 months) but in general the prognosis is excellent. Often, the course is more prolonged in adults or immunocompromised patients.

Hepatitis A infection does not have a carrier status. Progression to chronic viral disease does not occur, but in some individuals may precipitate autoimmune liver disease. Previous infection confers lifetime immunity.

Aims and indication for treatment

Unless the patient is very unwell, hospital admission is unnecessary. Treatment otherwise is supportive.

Vaccination or hyperimmune globulin should be offered to people at high risk.

Treatment

Antiemetics can be given for nausea and vomiting, intravenous fluids for dehydration, and simple analgesia for headaches. It is important to maintain caloric intake. Alcohol should be avoided.

Hepatitis B

Incidence

The symptomless infected carrier rate is 0.1% in the UK and USA, and 20% in parts of Asia and Africa (worldwide prevalence of carriers estimated at 300–400 million).

Transmission

- Contaminated blood products (incidence has fallen dramatically since the introduction of screening in the UK, Europe and the USA in the late 1970s and, subsequently, around the world, with the WHO vaccination programme).
- Contaminated instrumentation (intravenous drug user (IVDU)).
- Sexual intercourse with an infected partner.
- Vertical transmission (most common mode worldwide).
- Viral particles have been isolated from insects such as mosquitoes.

Aetiology and pathogenesis

Hepatitis B virus (HBV) is a DNA virus that replicates in the liver where the core antigen incorporates itself into the host genome. The host's DNA polymerase then transcribes for the virus. Viral DNA transcription products have been implicated in the development of hepatocellular carcinoma.

Body fluid contact is a prerequisite for transmission. Infection in the birth canal during parturition (vertical transmission) is the most important mode worldwide, creating a large 'carrier state' reservoir of infection. In developed countries, promiscuous sexual practitioners and IVDUs form the largest reservoir of infection.

Hepatitis B syndromes may be acute, chronic or the carrier state.

Clinical features

Features of acute hepatitis B:

- Incubation time: 60–160 days (average 90 days).
- Non-specific prodromal symptoms: arthralgia, anorexia, abdominal discomfort.
- Jaundice, fever and hepatomegaly are usual features.
- Urticarial or maculopapular rash may appear, together with a polyarthritis thought to be secondary to immune-mediated complexes.
- History of contact with a contaminated source is usual (especially travellers to the Orient, drug addicts, accidental injury to health workers, etc.).

Features of chronic hepatitis B:

- Most chronic carriers are asymptomatic.
- The majority are discovered incidentally (e.g. blood donor screening, occupational health checks, routine liver function tests, etc.).
- Patients with chronic active hepatitis may present with features or complications of chronic liver disease or cirrhosis: jaundice, ascites, portal hypertension, hepatic failure.
- Chronic hepatitis predisposes to cirrhosis of the liver and an increased risk of hepatocellular carcinoma, especially in males.

Diagnosis and investigations

Transaminases may be very high in the acute stage (1000–5000 IU/L) falling rapidly after the first week; chronic hepatitis produces only a mild elevation of ALT or AST.

Serology

Surface antigen (HBsAg) is the first serological marker to appear (6 weeks to 3 months); 'e' antigen (HBeAg) follows, reflecting viral replication, high infectivity and more severe disease. This usually disappears before HBsAg, but its persistence correlates with HBV

In chronic infection, the symptoms may persist for several months with bouts of fever and splenomegaly. Chronic derangements of liver biochemistry may be seen.

Diagnosis and investigation

Investigations to consider:

- Blood cultures are positive during acute infections in approximately half of patients. Rising titres are diagnostic.
- Liver biopsy may reveal presence of granulomas, but these are non-specific for brucellosis.

Aetiology and pathogenesis

A zoonosis due to a coccobacillus largely spread by ingestion of unpasteurized milk. Three species are recognized: *Brucella abortus* (cattle), *Brucella melitensis* (goats and sheep) and *Brucella suis* (pigs).

The organism travels via the lymphatics and infects lymph nodes and reticuloendothelial systems. Hypersensitivity may account for the formation of granulomas.

Treatment

A prolonged course of tetracycline and rifampicin is given. Alternatively, co-trimoxazole can be used.

METABOLIC AND GENETIC LIVER DISEASE

Haemochromatosis

Incidence

An autosomal recessive disorder due to excess iron accumulation affecting approximately 0.5% of the Caucasian population, with a heterozygote frequency of up to 10%.

Clinical features

Features are dependent on gender, dietary intake, age and associated toxins (e.g. alcohol) (Fig. 18.7). Women tend to present up to a decade later than men due to the protective mechanism of menstrual blood loss. In developing countries, iron deficiency and hookworm infestation can also delay manifestation of organ damage.

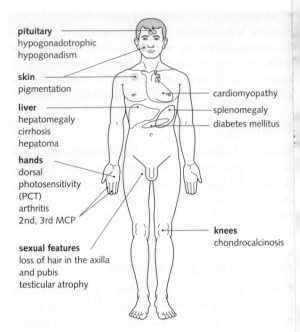

Fig. 18.7 Body map for haemochromatosis. (MCP, metacarpophalangeal joint; PCT, porphyria cutanea tarda.)

Patients may rarely present between the fourth and fifth decade with the classic triad of:

- Skin pigmentation (melanin deposition).
- Diabetes mellitus ('bronze diabetes').
- Hepatomegaly if the iron deposition is severe.

Other common presentations include gonadal atrophy and loss of libido secondary to pituitary dysfunction, cardiac failure, arthritis in the small joints of the hand and chondrocalcinosis in the knees.

Diagnosis and investigation

Investigations:

- Serum iron—usually elevated with a low total iron binding capacity.
- Transferrin saturation—grossly elevated (often 100%; normal <50%) but levels can also be moderately raised in heterozygotes.
- Serum ferritin—usually grossly elevated (>1000 µg/L; normal <300 males, <200 females). Ferritin can also be elevated in rheumatoid or other inflammatory diseases as it is an acute-phase protein, or in alcoholic liver disease, diabetes or the other metabolic diseases due to increased secretion. This occasionally causes confusion (see below).

- Liver biopsy confirms iron deposition and also provides an assessment of the extent of liver damage. Increased parenchymal iron deposition is also seen in alcoholic cirrhosis. Iron is demonstrated by Perl's potassium cyanide stain producing a Prussian blue appearance if haemosiderin iron is present. Iron deposition is graded I–IV depending on degree and distribution. Grades III and IV are usually diagnostic of haemochromatosis. A hepatic iron index of >1.9 (mg iron per mg dry weight liver divided by the patient's age in years) is also diagnostic and is useful for differentiating genetic haemochromatosis from iron loading in alcoholic liver disease.
- Fasting blood glucose should be taken to exclude secondary diabetes mellitus.
- An electrocardiogram should be undertaken to detect evidence of cardiomyopathy.
- The haemochromatosis gene, called HFE, has been identified. Genetic testing for the two major mutations (C282Y and H63D) is used in diagnosis.

Aetiology and pathogenesis

In the normal physiological state, iron absorption is regulated in the proximal small intestine according to the body's requirements. In haemochromatosis, the regulatory mechanism is faulty, leading to inappropriate levels of absorption even when iron stores are excessive.

The condition is characterized by increased deposition in the liver parenchymal cells in which extensive pigmentation and fibrosis develops and eventually cirrhosis occurs.

Increased iron content also occurs in endocrine glands, the heart and skin.

Iron accumulation is gradual throughout life and there is a threshold below which tissue damage may not occur (e.g. 5 mg/g in the liver), hence the late presentation.

There is an association with HLA-A3, B14 and B7 groups. The C282Y and H63D mutations in the HFE gene are responsible for almost all primary haemochromatosis.

Complications

If untreated, cirrhosis is a common end point followed by liver failure, which may be accompanied by portal hypertension.

Up to one-third of male patients who have cirrhosis may develop hepatocellular carcinoma.

Treating patients reverses the tissue damage and improves the survival rate (Fig. 18.8). However, the risk of malignant change may persist if cirrhosis is already present.

It is imperative to screen first-degree relatives for the condition before the development of irreversible liver damage. This can be achieved by checking serum ferritin levels or by attempting to identify the culpable gene. Genetic testing is more useful in first-degree relatives to predict risk even if ferritin is normal. Genetic testing for other subgroups has not been widely adopted because, although the condition tends to run 'true' in families, the phenotypic expression of the homozygous state in the wider population is variable (i.e. only a proportion of people homozygous for the mutation will develop iron overload). Biochemical testing with serum ferritin or transferrin saturation is more usually employed for screening the population.

Aims and indications for treatment

To reduce body iron stores (reflected by serum ferritin) to within normal levels and limit the progression of liver damage and other affected

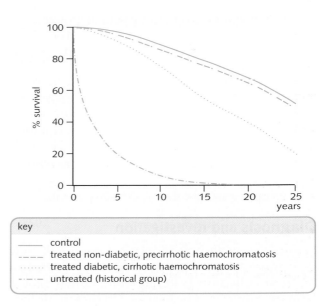

key

- —— control
- ---- treated non-diabetic, precirrhotic haemochromatosis
- .... treated diabetic, cirrhotic haemochromatosis
- -·-·- untreated (historical group)

Fig. 18.8 Survival with iron overload depends on the development of complications. Even so, depletion of iron stores prolongs survival. Life expectancy is normal if treatment is started before the onset of end-organ damage.

- Liver biopsy—piecemeal necrosis of chronic active hepatitis.
- Autoantibodies—positive anti-smooth muscle antibodies (present in 60%) (Fig. 18.15).

Aetiology and pathogenesis

Unknown cause. Thought to be immune mediated because there are abnormalities in T suppressor cells which may result from autoantibody production against hepatocyte antigens. A polyclonal elevation of IgG suggests defects in humoral response.

Association with other autoimmune disease (e.g. pernicious anaemia, systemic lupus erythematosus, thyroid disease, etc.) suggests cell-mediated response to own tissues. Lupus erythematosus (LE) cells are found in a number of liver biopsies, hence the old term 'lupoid hepatitis', but this confusing term should be avoided.

A number of drugs (e.g. methyldopa, ketoconazole, isoniazid) may cause a chronic hepatitis similar to the autoimmune variety and in some cases are related to acetylation of the drug by the liver. Autosomal genes influence a person's acetylator status, with the 'rapid' allele being dominant to the 'slow' allele. Homozygotes for the 'slow' allele have lower levels of the enzyme N-acetyltransferase in the liver. 'Slow' acetylators are at an increased risk of developing chronic active hepatitis compared with 'fast' acetylators.

Complications

Cirrhosis and liver failure. Patients are also more likely to develop other organ-specific autoimmune diseases.

Prognosis

A pattern of remission and exacerbation for several years followed by cirrhosis is characteristic. Half will die within 5 years if no treatment is given, compared with a 90% survival rate with treatment.

Aims and indications for treatment

Early diagnosis and prompt treatment are paramount in order to lessen the risk of mortality and morbidity.

Treatment plan

Corticosteroids to induce biochemical and histological remission, with subsequent addition of azathioprine (an antiproliferative immunosuppressant) as a steroid-sparing agent is the adopted treatment strategy.

Sarcoidosis and liver

Sarcoidosis is a chronic, multisystem disease characterized by the presence of non-caseating granulomas which predominantly affect the lung, lymph nodes and the skin, but the liver is also rarely affected. Cardiac, renal and neurological manifestations are also seen.

The underlying aetiology is unknown and the majority of cases present as an incidental finding of bilateral hilar lymphadenopathy.

It is a rare cause of hepatosplenomegaly, by producing portal hypertension either as a direct consequence of the granulomas compressing the portal venules or periportal scarring resulting in obstruction.

In cases of difficulty in diagnosing systemic sarcoidosis, a liver biopsy may be diagnostic especially in the presence of abnormal liver enzymes. Serum angiotensin-converting enzyme is often elevated, but not diagnostic, and more useful in monitoring disease activity. A Kveim skin test (still rarely performed by dermatologists) is positive.

Interpretation of autoantibody tests in liver disease					
Antibody	Inference	ALT, AST elevation	Alk Phos, GGT elevation	Raised immunoglobulins	Diagnostic test
AMA	PBC	Slight	Moderate	Mainly IgM, some IgG	AMA-M$_2$ subtype, liver biopsy
SMA, ANA, LKM	AICAH	Moderate	Slight	Mainly IgG	Liver biopsy
pANCA	PSC	Slight	Moderate	Some IgG	MRCP

Fig. 18.15 Comparison of antibody profiles in autoimmune liver disease. (AICAH, autoimmune chronic active hepatitis; ALT, alanine aminotransferase; Alk Phos, alkaline phosphatase; AMA, antimitochondrial antibody; ANA, antinuclear antibody; AST, Aspartate aminotransferase; MRCP, magnetic resonance cholangiopancreatography; GGT, gamma-glutamyl transferase; LKM, liver-kidney microsomal antibody; pANCA, perinuclear anti-neutrophil cytoplasmic antibody; PBC, primary biliary cirrhosis; PSC, primary sclerosing cholangitis; SMA, smooth muscle antibody.)

Hepatic complications are those of portal hypertension with or without decompensated liver disease.

Treatment is with systemic steroids to induce remission of the disease. Methotrexate and azathioprine are sometimes used as steroid-sparing agents for protracted therapy or refractory disease, but the long-term benefit is currently unclear.

Alcoholic liver disease

Incidence and diagnosis

Approximately 1% of the population are psychologically or physically dependent upon alcohol:

- 20–30% of these develop alcoholic liver disease.
- Approximately 25% of liver cirrhosis is due to alcohol.

Current recommendations for safe alcohol consumption: 21 (male) and 14 (female) units per week:

- A unit of alcohol (approximately 10 g) represents a measure of spirit, half a glass of wine or half a pint of beer (see Fig. 21.3).
- An intake of 20 units (or more) per day is associated with a high risk of hepatocellular damage.

Obtaining a history of excessive alcohol use is not always straightforward. Patients may well deny excessive use and often under-report the actual amount they drink. The family of a patient who becomes unwell from complications of their alcoholic liver disease sometimes harbour feelings of guilt at being unable to alter the drinking behaviour of a loved one. It is helpful to acknowledge the difficulties and frustrations of a family coping with alcoholism.

Clinical features

Diagnosis is made predominantly on clinical grounds, and the extent of liver damage can be determined by liver biopsy but does not always correlate well with deranged liver biochemistry.

Symptoms can often be vague, including nausea, vomiting, abdominal pain and diarrhoea; and may be attributable to the effects of alcohol or alcohol withdrawal per se. More extensive hepatocellular damage may manifest from jaundice to hepatic failure.

Extra-hepatic manifestations include:

- Wernicke's encephalopathy (confusion, nystagmus, ataxia, ophthalmoplegia) and Korsakoff's psychosis (short-term memory loss).
- Proximal myopathy.
- Peripheral neuropathy (often painful).
- Cardiomyopathy, with cardiac failure and arrythmias.
- Gastritis and erosions.
- Porphyria cutanea tarda.
- Neglect and malnutrition.
- Psychosocial difficulties.

The CAGE questionnaire is a quick assessment for evidence of dependency on alcohol. Ask the patient whether they have ever:

- **C**ut down on alcohol for any reason.
- Become **A**ngry when people discuss their alcohol consumption.
- Felt **G**uilty because of their alcohol consumption.
- Needed an **E**ye opener early in the day to help them cope.

Don't forget to ask about past alcohol use as well as current drinking patterns. The effect of previous excessive alcohol intake may only become apparent years later as symptoms of liver disease appear.

Pathogenesis

Three main types of liver damage are described:

1. Fatty change.
2. Alcoholic hepatitis.
3. Fibrosis.

Fatty change

Ethanol is metabolized in the liver, which results in hepatic fatty acid synthesis and reduced fatty acid oxidation leading to accumulation and fatty destruction of the hepatic cells (Fig. 18.16). Similar changes can also be seen in obesity, diabetes, starvation, and pregnancy.

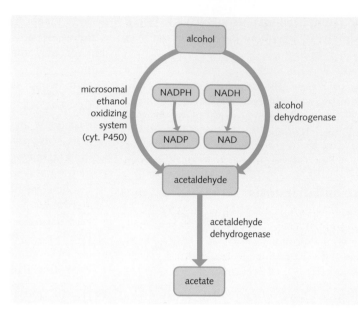

Fig. 18.16 Biochemical pathways for metabolism of alcohol. Alcohol under normal circumstances is converted to acetaldehyde by the action of alcohol dehydrogenase. In heavy drinkers, induction of the cytochrome P450 enzyme system occurs, hence increasing the metabolism of alcohol. Free radicals are a by-product of NADP and NAD production causing hepatocellular damage.

There is thought to be no permanent hepatocellular damage, hence fatty change resolves with abstinence from alcohol.

Alcoholic hepatitis

Infiltration with polymorphonuclear leucocytes and hyaline material (Mallory bodies) is typical. Fatty change often coexists with alcoholic hepatitis. Mallory bodies may also be seen in this form of chronic active hepatitis; they are not specific to alcoholic damage.

Fibrosis

Characterized by fibrosis with nodular regeneration which implies previous or continuing liver damage. A micronodular pattern progresses to macronodular in later stages.

Diagnosis and investigation

A background of chronic liver disease and a history of heavy alcohol consumption are highly indicative of alcoholic liver disease.

Other investigations may aid diagnosis:

- FBC—often reveals a macrocytosis (a sensitive indicator of heavy alcohol consumption). Leucocytosis is common. Thrombocytopenia occurs as a result of the toxic effect of ethanol on megakaryocytes.
- Liver biochemistry: gamma-glutamyl transferase is another indicator of heavy alcohol intake. In the presence of hepatitis, raised AST, ALT, bilirubin and alkaline phosphatase will be seen. Aspartate aminotransferase is usually only moderately raised at levels below 300 IU/L; ALT is usually less than half that value and it has been suggested that the AST:ALT ratio is a useful indicator of alcoholic liver disease when in excess of 2. Low albumin may suggest underlying cirrhosis and impaired synthetic function. Associated hyperlipidaemia with haemolytic anaemia can occasionally be seen (Zieve syndrome).
- Clotting screen—prolonged prothrombin time is typical of alcoholic hepatitis due to reduced production of clotting factors by the liver.
- Ultrasound will demonstrate fatty change and, if there is macronodular cirrhosis, may demonstrate an irregular margin with irregular intra-hepatic foci mimicking metastatic disease.
- Liver biopsy is the gold standard for diagnosing alcoholic liver injury. Transjugular liver biopsy may be necessary to reduce the bleeding risk in patients with a coagulopathy and/or low platelet count. Features of fatty change and cirrhosis will be seen. End-stage cirrhosis seen on histology will not distinguish its underlying aetiology.

Complications

Liver failure and cirrhosis.

Prognosis

Dependent on abstinence. Patients without established cirrhosis have a 5-year survival of 60% if they continue to drink alcohol, which rises to 90%

if they discontinue. Cirrhotic patients who continue to drink alcohol have an even poorer prognosis with 5-year survival rate of 35%.

Treatment

Abstinence from alcohol is vital. Acute alcohol withdrawal (i.e. hallucinations, tremor, fits, delirium tremens) should be treated with a reducing regime of a benzodiazepine such as diazepam or chlordiazepoxide. Wernicke's encephalopathy is reversible and is treated as an emergency with intravenous thiamine (Pabrinex). High protein and calorie supplements should be given, except in cases of hepatic encephalopathy.

Treatment of cirrhosis is described below.

CIRRHOSIS

Cirrhosis is the end stage of any progressive liver disease.

Clinical features

Cirrhosis per se is usually asymptomatic. Symptoms arise either due to the underlying disease or when complications of cirrhosis ensue.

Abdominal examination may reveal:

- Hepatomegaly or splenomegaly (if portal hypertension is present).
- Ascites.
- Dilated umbilical veins (caput medusae; Fig. 18.17).

Stigmata of chronic liver disease in the skin include anaemia, jaundice, palmar erythema, Dupuytren's contracture, finger clubbing, leuconychia, pruritus, spider naevi and xanthomas.

There may be endocrine features, such as loss of hair, testicular atrophy, parotid enlargement, gynaecomastia, amenorrhoea and a loss of libido.

Neurological features include drowsiness, confusion, asterixis (flapping hand tremor), constructional apraxia and foetor hepaticus (portosystemic encephalopathy).

Fluid retention may be apparent in the abdomen (ascites) or as peripheral oedema.

Investigations

Investigations to consider include the following:

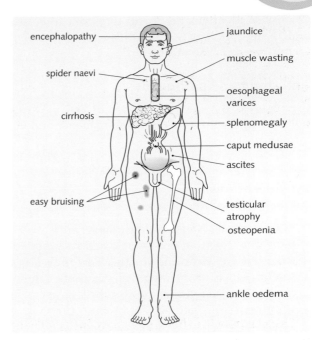

Fig. 18.17 Body map showing features of cirrhosis.

- Liver biochemistry can be surprisingly normal but some abnormality will often be present with slightly raised transaminases and alkaline phosphatase. In severe cases, all liver enzymes will be abnormal. Dilutional hyponatraemia and albumin are also seen. Hyperglycaemia can be evident if there is associated pancreatic insufficiency, and hypertriglyceridaemia is common.
- FBC may reveal anaemia. Macrocytosis can be a direct effect of alcohol in addition to vitamin B_{12} or folate deficiency.
- Coagulopathy is a very sensitive indicator of liver dysfunction and is reflected in the prolonged prothrombin time.
- Alpha-fetoprotein is raised in hepatocellular carcinoma (although can be slightly elevated with cirrhosis—serial measurements are useful).
- Ultrasound provides information on liver size, fatty change and fibrosis as well as hepatocellular carcinoma.
- Endoscopy identifies and allows treatment for varices.
- Liver biopsy establishes the diagnosis of cirrhosis. It may be indicated for patients in whom the underlying aetiology is unclear or to assess the severity of cirrhosis.

Other investigations are useful in establishing the underlying aetiology (e.g. hepatitis serology, ferritin, caeruloplasmin, autoantibodies).

Aetiology and pathogenesis

Cirrhosis of the liver is a result of cell necrosis followed by fibrosis and regeneration, hence nodule formation (Fig. 18.18).

The most common cause worldwide is chronic hepatitis B infection, whereas in the Western world, alcohol is the culprit.

Two types of cirrhosis have been described:

1. Macronodular—regenerating nodules are generally larger and of a variable size. They are often a result of chronic hepatitis B or C infection.
2. Micronodular—contains nodules that are <3 mm in size, uniformly affects the liver and is more often seen with ongoing alcohol abuse. However, a mixed picture can be seen and the underlying cause does not necessarily reflect the histological change.

Complications

Portal hypertension

Portal vascular resistance is increased due to collagen deposition and fibrosis seen in liver cirrhosis and, hence, formation of varices in the gastro-oesophageal junction (Fig. 18.19). In addition, sodium retention and vasoactive substances such as nitric oxide (due to accumulation of toxic metabolites) will increase plasma volume and splanchnic vasodilatation respectively, and thus maintain portal hypertension.

Bleeding from varices will result in haematemesis and melaena and can be precipitated by trauma (e.g. food bolus) or rising portal venous pressure (i.e. progressive liver cirrhosis).

Ascites

This is a result of fluid in the peritoneal cavity, and its pathogenesis involves several physiological processes.

Sodium and water retention occur as a result of activation of the renin–angiotensin system, secondary to arterial vasodilatation (caused by vasoactive substances such as nitric oxide). Portal hypertension per se results in a transudative ascites due to increased hydrostatic pressure, hence it further reduces intravascular volume and stimulates sodium and water retention via aldosterone (secondary hyperaldosteronism).

Ascites may be aggravated by a low plasma oncotic pressure resulting from hypoalbuminaemia, which occurs as a result of impaired synthetic hepatic function.

Spontaneous infection of ascites (spontaneous bacterial peritonitis (SBP)) is a serious complication:

- Affects 15% of patients admitted with ascites.
- Mortality is 20% if detected and treated promptly.

Patients are frequently asymptomatic and there should be a high index of suspicion. Spontaneous bacterial peritonitis should be excluded if the following occur:

- Nausea, mild abdominal pain and vomiting.
- Non-specific clinical deterioration.
- Fever, neutrophilia.

Ascitic fluid should be aspirated for culture and cell count. Ascitic fluid should be inoculated into blood

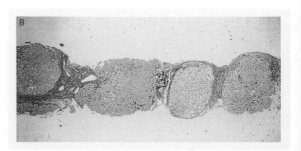

A	Causes of cirrhosis
Alcohol excess	
Chronic viral hepatitis, especially B and C	
Genetic diseases, e.g. haemochromatosis, alpha-1-antitrypsin deficiency	
Chronic liver diseases, e.g. primary biliary cirrhosis, chronic active hepatitis	
Cryptogenic where no aetiology is apparent but the patient presents with complications	

Fig. 18.18 (A) Common causes of cirrhosis. (B) Low-power photomicrograph of needle liver biopsy showing fibrous nodular formation and established cirrhosis.

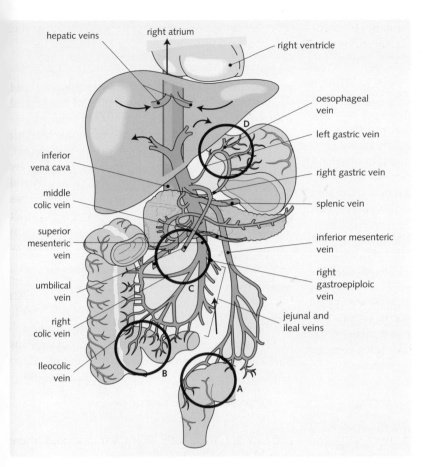

Fig. 18.19 Portal vasculature and sites of portal systemic anastomoses. Sites of portosystemic anastomoses are indicated by black circles. (A) Rectal varices or haemorrhoids. (B) Ileocaecal varices. (C) Umbilical varices (caput medusae). (D) Gastro-oesophageal varices. Varices at the gastro-oesophageal junction bleed most commonly only because they traverse the greatest pressure gradient between the negative pressure in the thorax and the positive-pressure abdominal cavity.

culture bottles. Treatment with a fluoroquinolone (e.g. ciprofloxacin) or a third-generation cephalosporin (e.g. cefotaxime) should be employed.

Hepatic encephalopathy

Toxic metabolites that are usually detoxified by the liver accumulate in the bloodstream and pass through the blood–brain barrier to cause encephalopathy. Ammonia produced by the breakdown of proteins by intestinal bacteria appears to play a role in hepatic encephalopathy. Accumulation of false neurotransmitters is also important, though poorly understood.

Clinically, the patient is confused, disorientated, has slurred speech and, in severe cases, convulsion and coma. Coarse flapping of hyperextended hands (asterixis), hepatic fetor (sweet-smelling breath due to ketones) and constructional apraxia (unable to draw a five-pointed star) can also be seen.

Acute onset usually has a precipitating factor which potentially can be reversible (e.g. bleeding, infection or constipation).

Hepatorenal syndrome

Characterized by cirrhosis, jaundice and renal failure.

It is thought to be due to a depletion in intravascular volume, activation of the renin–angiotensin system and vasoconstriction of the renal afferent arterioles, hence reduced glomerular filtration.

Other mediators have also been implicated that are related to prostaglandin synthesis, and the syndrome can be precipitated by the use of non-steroidal anti-inflammatory drugs (NSAIDs). More commonly, renal impairment occurs as a result of sepsis, diuretic use or excessive paracentesis causing intravascular volume depletion and renal hypoperfusion.

The renal abnormality is thought to be functional because transplanted kidneys from a donor patient with hepatorenal syndrome to a recipient will result in a normal functioning kidney. However, extreme cases will cause tubular necrosis and renal damage.

The patient should be treated for pre-renal failure but the condition carries a very high mortality.

Hepatocellular carcinoma

Development of cirrhosis is an independent risk factor for hepatocellular carcinoma (see Tumours of the liver, below).

Prognosis

Grading of prognosis of cirrhosis is made on the Child's criteria (Fig. 18.20). Overall, there is a 50% survival in 5 years.

Treatment

Generally consists of managing the complications that arise.

If ascites is present, spontaneous bacterial infection must be excluded and, if found, appropriate therapy should be started.

A reduction in dietary sodium will allow the reabsorption of ascitic fluid back into the circulation.

Diuretic therapy is used to increase renal excretion of sodium and hence excess water. Hepatic dysfunction results in secondary hyperaldosteronism because of failure to break down aldosterone in the liver. Spironolactone, a specific aldosterone antagonist, is therefore the diuretic of choice. If the maximum dose of spironolactone is ineffective, a loop diuretic such as furosemide can be used, but the patient is at risk of hyponatraemia, dehydration and hypokalaemia. Paracentesis is often carried out for symptomatic relief (up to 20 L can be drained).

Hypovolaemia is problematic because ascites reaccumulates at the expense of circulating volume. This can be avoided by administration of salt-poor albumin or plasma expanders such as gelofusin.

Various shunts can be inserted for persistent ascites such that they drain peritoneal fluid into the internal jugular vein, but infection and blockage of the shunts limit their use. Intra-hepatic shunts (TIPS, see below) can be used for refractory ascites.

For hepatic encephalopathy, an underlying precipitating cause should be found and appropriate treatment instigated (i.e. correction of electrolyte imbalance, treatment of sepsis, etc.). Laxatives and enemas should be given to reduce ammonia load.

Oesophageal and gastric varices

Incidence

Major complication of cirrhosis, whatever the underlying aetiology. Up to 70% of cirrhotic patients will develop varices and up to 40% of these will bleed.

Portal vein thrombosis causes non-cirrhotic portal hypertension.

Clinical features

Acute GI bleed in the form of melaena or haematemesis due to rupture of varices is the usual mode of presentation. Other features may include:

- Stigmata of chronic liver disease—palmar erythema, spider naevi, proximal myopathy or muscle wasting, pigmentation or jaundice, hypogonadism.
- Splenomegaly—usually present due to underlying portal hypertension.
- Features of liver failure (e.g. encephalopathy, ascites, jaundice, etc.).

Diagnosis and investigation

- FBC, biochemistry, clotting, etc., as for all patients with an acute GI bleed. A low

Fig. 18.20 Modified Child classification of cirrhosis based on functional capacity of the liver. Class C carries a poor prognosis.

	Modified Child classification		
Child's class	A	B	C
Serum bilirubin µmol/L	Normal	Up to twice normal	More than twice normal
Serum albumin g/L	Normal	30–35	Less than 30 g/L
Ascites	None	Minimal and responds to diuretics	Moderate or marked
Encephalopathy	None	None or mild irritability	Grades II, III, IV
Coagulopathy	None	Prothrombin time ≤4 s prolonged	PT ≥5 s prolonged

platelet count may indicate hypersplenism due to portal hypertension. Prolonged prothrombin time is an indicator of diminished hepatic synthetic function.

- Urgent endoscopy is essential to confirm the diagnosis and differentiate variceal haemorrhage from other causes.
- Liver biopsy may be required, following recovery from the acute episode, if the aetiology of liver disease remains in doubt.
- Ultrasound and Doppler studies may be useful to diagnose hepatic or portal vein thrombosis.

Aetiology and pathogenesis

Due to presence of portal hypertension, which can be:

- Pre-sinusoidal.
- Sinusoidal.
- Post-sinusoidal.

When portal pressure rises above 10–12 mmHg (normal = 5–8 mmHg), collateral communication with the systemic venous system occurs instead of blood flowing into the hepatic vein. Portosystemic anastomoses occur at the gastro-oesophageal junction, ileocaecal junction, rectum and anterior abdominal wall via the umbilical vein (Figs. 18.19 and 18.21).

Pre-sinusoidal

This is blockage of the portal vein before its entry to the liver (e.g. portal vein thrombosis as a result of congenital venous abnormality, prothrombotic states or umbilical sepsis). Pancreatic disease is the most common cause in adults. A rare cause is schistosomiasis. Doppler studies usually identify the blockage.

Sinusoidal

The majority of cases are due to cirrhosis, where portal vascular resistance is increased due to distorted architecture and perivenular fibrosis. This can also occur in congenital hepatic fibrosis and non-cirrhotic portal hypertension, where the histology shows mild portal tract fibrosis without cirrhosis.

Post-sinusoidal

Budd–Chiari syndrome where there is occlusion of the hepatic veins as they exit the liver. The patient usually has a hypercoagulable state, underlying myeloproliferative disorder or extrinsic occlusion by a tumour or mass.

Portal hypertension develops if the condition becomes chronic. Other causes include constrictive pericarditis and right-sided cardiac failure.

Complications

Risk of developing encephalopathy is high with an acute variceal bleed.

Prognosis

Overall risk of recurrence after an acute episode is 80% over 2 years. Each variceal bleed carries a mortality risk of 15–40%.

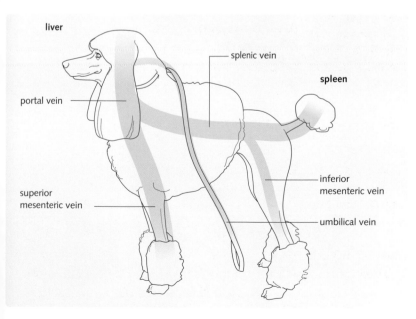

Fig. 18.21 Difficulty remembering the portal circulation? For portal, think poodle!

Aims of treatment

Resuscitation, restoration of haemodynamic stability and arrest of variceal bleeding. Once this is successfully carried out, then preventive measures should be started.

Treatment

Resuscitation aims to replace depleted intravascular volume with plasma expanders and crystalloids initially, then blood once available (as with all major GI bleeds). Correction of coagulopathy with vitamin K (takes 6–12 hours to work), fresh frozen plasma or cryoprecipitate should be undertaken if required. A vasopressin analogue, e.g. terlipressin, can be administered intravenously as an adjuvant therapy. The aim is to cause splanchnic vasoconstriction and hence restrict portal blood flow. Antibiotic treatment improves survival in patients with variceal bleeding.

Urgent endoscopy is required. Sclerosant is injected in or around the varices to cause inflammatory obliteration. Alternatively, elastic band ligation of the varices at endoscopy produces thrombotic

obliteration (Fig. 18.22). Repeat sclerotherapy or banding is usually employed to eradicate varices with the intention of preventing further bleeds.

Balloon tamponade is mainly reserved for patients for whom endoscopic therapy is temporarily unavailable or the procedure has failed. An inflatable tube is passed into the stomach and the balloon inflated with air. Traction on the balloon is maintained for 12 hours. An alternative design of tube also has an oesophageal balloon. Prolonged inflation of the balloon is associated with mucosal ulceration and rupture of the oesophagus. It also increases the risk of aspiration pneumonia.

Transjugular intra-hepatic portosystemic shunt (TIPS) is a shunt formed between the systemic and portal venous system to treat varices (Fig. 18.23). A guidewire is passed under X-ray control via the internal jugular vein to the hepatic vein and passes into the liver. Contact is made through the liver substance with the portal venous circulation and a metal endoprosthesis is inserted to create the shunt. Encephalopathy occurs in up to 30% patients. Recurrence of varices can occur if the stent thromboses.

Fig. 18.22 Strategy to control variceal haemorrhage by elastic band ligation.

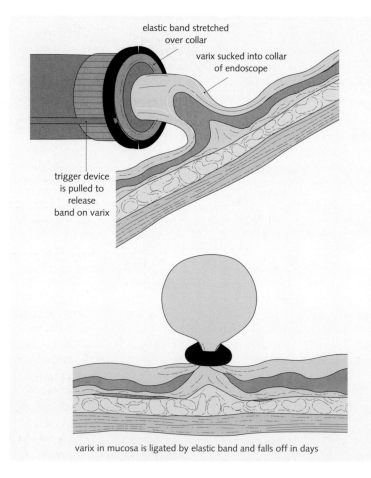

elastic band stretched over collar

varix sucked into collar of endoscope

trigger device is pulled to release band on varix

varix in mucosa is ligated by elastic band and falls off in days

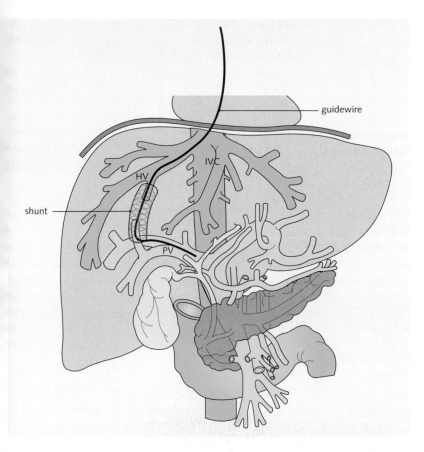

Surgery is rarely performed nowadays. Oesophageal transection can be done as an emergency with ligation of the vessels. Portosystemic shunts (mesocaval or splenorenal) can also be undertaken surgically but have a high incidence of encephalopathy. Narrow gauge stents forming a conduit between the portal vein and vena cava can improve the results but have no advantage over TIPS.

A non-selective beta-blocker (e.g. propranolol) can be given to reduce portal pressure by reducing cardiac output and allowing vasoconstriction of splanchnic arteries by inhibiting the effects of β_2 receptor-mediated vasodilatation. This is the drug of choice in both primary prevention of variceal bleeding and in prevention of secondary haemorrhage following obliteration of varices. Patients with varices that have not bled are given propranolol as primary prophylaxis against bleeding.

TUMOURS OF THE LIVER

The most common tumours are metastatic spread from another primary site (e.g. GI tract, breast, thyroid and bronchus). Primary tumours of the liver are usually malignant.

Hepatocellular carcinoma

Incidence

One of the most common malignant diseases worldwide but rare in the Western world.

Clinical features

- Usually non-specific (i.e. weight loss, malaise, fever, right upper quadrant pain) and, in late stages, ascites (an exudate, that may be bloodstained).
- Cirrhotic patients who develop the above clinical features should have malignant change excluded.
- An enlarged irregular tender liver is more likely to be found in secondary metastasis or pre-existing cirrhosis than primary hepatocellular carcinoma.
- Metastases to lung and bone may produce pleural effusions and pathological fractures, respectively.

Diagnosis and investigation

Investigations to consider:

- Liver biochemistry—normal or mild abnormality of enzymes is usual in established, inactive cirrhosis. A rise in ALT or AST may be indicative of tumour necrosis. Elevated alkaline phosphatase may reflect bony metastases.
- Serum alpha-fetoprotein raised in 80% (often normal in small tumours).
- Liver ultrasound will identify majority of liver tumours.
- Computed tomography (CT) or magnetic resonance imaging (MRI) are also useful imaging modalities.
- Cytology of ascitic fluid may demonstrate malignant cells.
- Liver biopsy under ultrasound guidance is rarely required for histological diagnosis. Tumour may seed down the biopsy track and biopsy is avoided if potentially curative surgery can be offered.
- Six-monthly ultrasound scan and alpha-fetoprotein are offered to patients with liver cirrhosis as surveillance for hepatoma.

Aetiology and pathogenesis

In areas where hepatitis B and C are prevalent, over 90% of patients with hepatocellular carcinoma have positive serology and an equal number have pre-existing cirrhosis. The aetiology is presumed to be the integration of the virus into the host genome.

Most patients with cirrhosis, whatever the underlying cause, are at risk of developing hepatocellular carcinoma, but especially patients with hepatitis B and primary haemochromatosis. Development of a hepatoma occurs more commonly in males than females with cirrhosis.

Prognosis

Very poor: <5% survival at 6 months.

Treatment

Little response to radiotherapy or chemotherapy. Isolated lesions may be surgically resected. A patient with cirrhosis and a small tumour may be offered transplantation.

Other tumours of the liver

Adenomas

Rare—associated with the oral contraceptive pill. Can present as an incidental finding or due to intra-hepatic bleeding. Surgical resection is considered for larger adenomas because of the risk of rupture or malignant transformation. The oral contraceptive pill should be stopped.

Haemangiomas

Most common benign tumour of the liver and usually found incidentally on ultrasound. No treatment is required. If diagnosis is in doubt, then angiography is required.

Focal nodular hyperplasia

As its name suggests, this condition causes nodules in the liver, but hepatic function is normal. It is more common than hepatic adenoma but has no malignant potential. Its importance is that it can be mistaken for cirrhosis, either on radiological imaging or even on histology from a needle biopsy. It is usually asymptomatic and found incidentally, but is believed to be related to the oral contraceptive pill. In these circumstances, it is thought that about 50% become symptomatic, usually with pain in the right upper quadrant. Symptomatic cases are treated by surgical resection.

DRUGS AND THE LIVER

Many drugs are metabolized by liver enzymes and some are excreted in bile. Some drugs are fat soluble and their bioavailability can be affected by bile salt micellar concentration in the intestine. Plasma proteins, especially albumin synthesized in the liver, affect the kinetics of many drugs. Hence liver dysfunction and disease can impair absorption, transport, metabolism and excretion of several drugs (Fig. 18.24). Care must be taken when using most drugs in the presence of liver disease. Conversely, many drugs can cause deranged liver biochemistry or damage.

Drug toxicity to the liver

Incidence

Up to 10% of jaundice is drug induced and is mediated by different mechanisms.

Aetiology and pathogenesis

Drug toxicity can be:

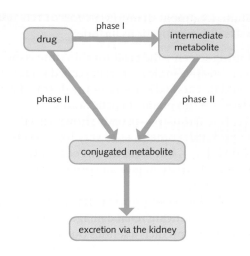

Fig. 18.24 Biochemical pathways of drug metabolism in the liver.

- Dose or duration related (e.g. azathioprine, methotrexate).
- Idiosyncratic (e.g. flucloxacillin, clavulanic acid).
- Due to overdose toxicity (e.g. paracetamol).

Three types of pathology are described (Fig. 18.25):

1. Acute hepatitis typically occurs 2–3 weeks after starting the drug and normally resolves after cessation.
2. Cholestasis—bile stasis causes a functional obstruction, hence biochemically it produces jaundice with pale stools and dark urine usually after 4–6 weeks. The cause of bile stasis is unclear but inflammatory infiltration of bile ducts and interference with excretory transport proteins have been implicated. Anabolic steroids and oral contraceptives can cause profound cholestasis.
3. Necrosis—mainly dose dependent. Toxic metabolites are normally detoxified by the liver (e.g. conjugation by glutathione), and once the level of glutathione falls, toxic metabolites accumulate and liver necrosis follows. Concurrent ingestion of enzyme-inducing drugs (e.g. phenytoin, carbamazepine, an alcohol binge), severely ill patients or starvation will render these individuals more susceptible to toxicity.

Clinical features

These can range from mild elevation of liver enzymes to acute fulminant hepatic failure:

- Jaundice is usually secondary to an acute hepatitis or cholestasis but rarely it can be due to haemolysis.
- In the majority of cases, derangement of liver enzymes is found on routine examination before clinical jaundice develops.
- Nausea and vomiting or abdominal pain may occur.
- Pruritus, steatorrhoea and dark urine are present if cholestasis occurs.

Diagnosis and investigation

Enquire carefully about the timing, chronology and duration of drug ingestion.

Drugs affecting liver function	
Pattern of liver damage	**Drugs**
Hepatitis	Antituberculous: rifampicin, isoniazid Antifungal: ketoconazole Antihypertensive: atenolol, verapamil Anaesthetics: halothane
Cholestasis	Antiarrhythmics: amiodarone Antimetabolite: methotrexate Allopurinol Antipsychotics: chlorpromazine Antibiotics: erythromycin, clavulanic acid, flucloxacillin Immunosuppressives: ciclosporin A Contraceptives and anabolic steroids
Necrosis	Paracetamol, carbon tetrachloride

Fig. 18.25 Drugs known to cause disturbance in liver function.

Courvoisier's sign—the presence of painless obstructive jaundice and a palpable gall bladder suggests that the cause is not gallstones. Gallstones tend to produce a fibrotic reaction in the gall bladder which then shrinks down.

Aetiology and pathogenesis

The aetiology is unknown but smoking and high alcohol consumption have been implicated. The role of chronic pancreatitis as a risk factor is uncertain as familial chronic pancreatitis is associated with a significantly increased risk of cancer.

Almost all tumours are due to adenocarcinoma arising from the duct epithelium and around 70% are in the head of the pancreas. The tumours have usually already metastasized to local lymph nodes and the liver by the time of presentation.

Prognosis

Very poor due to its late presentation. The 5-year survival is <5%.

Aims of treatment

This is mainly for palliation because curative treatment is uncommon due to the nature of the disease.

Treatment

Options include:

- Radical surgical resection—provides the only possible chance of a cure, but it is seldom carried out. Fewer than 30% of patients are resectable at the time of presentation and the operative mortality is about 5%. A bypass operation for the relief of jaundice can be performed where the common bile duct is anastomosed to the small bowel as a palliative measure.
- Stent insertion—can be achieved endoscopically or percutaneously where a stent is inserted into the narrowed part of the common bile duct to allow free drainage of bile.
- Analgesia in the form of opiates is indicated, as dependence is not an issue.

- Coeliac axis block may be useful for patients with pain that is not controlled by conventional analgesia.
- A variety of chemotherapeutic agents are used with variable efficacy.

ENDOCRINE TUMOURS

Incidence

These are rare tumours in the pancreas and can occur with tumours of the pituitary and parathyroid to form a syndrome of multiple endocrine neoplasia (MEN).

Clinical features

Depend on the cell type and the hormone produced.

Gastrinomas (Zollinger–Ellison syndrome)

These arise from the G cells of the pancreas and they secrete gastrin and present as peptic ulceration which is often large and multiple. Perforation and gastrointestinal haemorrhage are common and diagnosis should be considered in young patients presenting with recurrent peptic ulcer disease.

Diarrhoea due to excess acid production is also common.

Insulinomas (Islet cell tumours)

Produce insulin and present as episodes of fasting hypoglycaemia (i.e. early morning or late afternoon).

Presentation is often bizarre, hence diagnosis may not be made for years and the patient learns to live with the symptoms, as glucose abolishes the attacks.

VIPomas

These are rare pancreatic tumours in which vasoactive intestinal peptide (VIP) is produced, causing severe secretory diarrhoea, leading to dehydration by stimulating adenyl cyclase to produce intestinal secretions.

Glucagonomas

Tumours of alpha cells that produce glucagon in patients with diabetes mellitus. A characteristic rash (necrolytic migratory erythema) has also been described.

Somatostatinomas

Somatostatin is an inhibitory hormone that produces a reduction in the secretion of insulin, pancreatic enzyme and bicarbonate, hence producing the clinical syndrome of diabetes mellitus, steatorrhoea and hypochlorhydria.

Weight loss is also a common feature.

Diagnosis and investigation

This again is dependent on the type of tumour involved and the clinical presentation:

- A CT scan will identify the majority of endocrine tumours in the pancreas.
- Hormone assays—measurement of the specific type of hormone produced will often give the diagnosis. Selective venous sampling from the pancreas will also help to locate the tumour. In cases of insulinoma, measurement is usually made during a 24–48-hour fast when symptoms of hypoglycaemia appear.

Aetiology and pathogenesis

These are neuroendocrine tumours. The MEN type 2 syndrome has an autosomal dominant inheritance.

Prognosis

Gastrinomas are often malignant, hence carry a worse prognosis than insulinomas, which are benign. Overall prognosis will depend on associated MEN syndrome and other tumours involved.

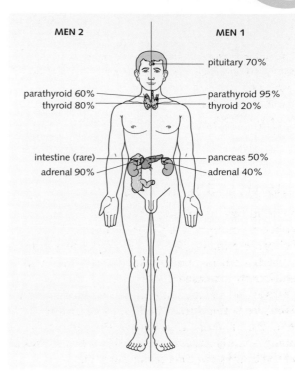

Fig. 20.9 Depiction of multiple endocrine neoplasia (MEN) 1 and MEN 2.

Treatment

Surgical resection of the tumour is required.

Identification of other possible tumours associated with MEN syndrome may be required and screening of relatives in those with MEN type 2 syndrome (Fig. 20.9).

HISTORY, EXAMINATION AND COMMON INVESTIGATIONS

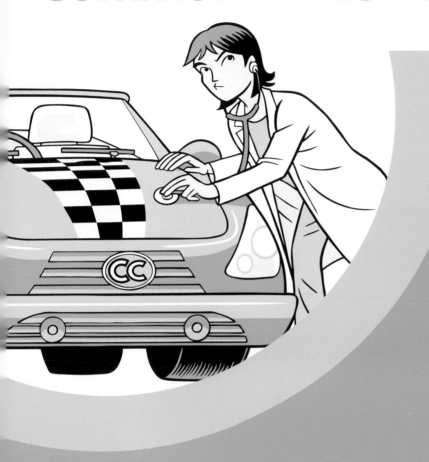

Objectives

You should be able to:

- Take a history from a patient—with specific relevance to symptoms arising from gastrointestinal disease
- Calculate the number of units of alcohol a patient drinks a week

Preliminaries

Introduce yourself, be polite, listen carefully and look interested, even if you have been up all night!

Give patients the time and the opportunity to tell you what you need to know, and put them at ease, as many symptoms are embarrassing.

Maintain eye contact (even if patients do not) and watch carefully for clues about how ill they look. Are they agitated, distressed or in pain? Is there a discernible tremor or involuntary movement? Is there evidence of significant weight loss (cachexia)? Do they have a pale, pigmented or jaundiced complexion?

Look around the bedside for clues (e.g. inhalers, oxygen, a walking stick or frame, cards from family and friends, sputum pots, reading material and glasses, special food preparations, etc.).

THE STANDARD STRUCTURE OF A HISTORY

It is important to maintain a structured approach to your history taking, particularly in the early stages of your career. You are less likely to omit relevant questions if your history is structured. It is preferable to commit the format to memory, and acquire the relevant information in conversational form, so that constant reference to notes is avoided during the interaction.

The purpose of taking a history is to arrive at a differential diagnosis. Some information is background and may not be immediately obvious or useful, but can often be vital later on.

Description of the patient

This should include brief demographic details, including the patient's age, sex, ethnic origins and occupation. It should allow others who have not met the patient to picture him or her in their mind.

Presenting complaint

What prompted the patient to seek help? This will usually be a specific or particular symptom, but may be difficult to identify immediately. Your task is to focus on the symptoms and crystallize them into problems that can be addressed.

Note down the sites of pain (Fig. 21.1).

History of presenting complaint

This is a complete description of the problem that brought the patient to see you:

- How and when the symptoms started.
- The speed of onset—was it rapid, or slow and insidious?

Fig. 21.1 Sites of pain and possible significance. (GORD, gastro-oesophageal reflux disease.)

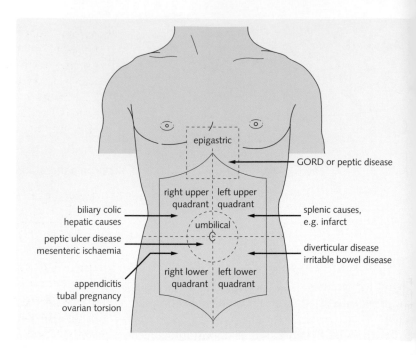

- The pattern of symptoms, their duration and frequency—are they continuous or intermittent? How often do they appear?
- If the symptoms include pain, you should describe it comprehensively! Relevant features are onset, site, severity, character (sharp, crushing, gnawing, etc.), radiation, frequency, periodicity, associated features, precipitating and relieving factors, relationship to meals, posture and alcohol.
- Why has the patient decided to consult the doctor at this juncture? What is different?
- Find out the extent of any deficit. Is there any loss of function, anything specific the patient cannot do or any impact on their lifestyle?
- Is there anything else the patient thinks may be relevant, however trivial?

Past medical history

Has the patient had any medical or surgical contact in the past? Ask specifically about operations, previous transfusions, drugs, especially antibiotics, allergies and previous investigations.

Obstetric and menstrual history should also be recorded.

Drug history

Ask about all drugs, including contraceptive pills and over-the-counter medicines, as well as medicines that have been prescribed.

Non-steroidal anti-inflammatory drugs are commonly taken as over-the-counter medicines and can cause ulcers.

It may be necessary to contact family members or the general practitioner to establish an accurate list of the patient's current prescribed therapy.

It is common for a patient to profess to having a drug allergy, when in fact an adverse side effect has occurred (e.g. diarrhoea after taking penicillin or dyspepsia with aspirin). It is important to establish whether they are truly allergic to a particular drug, as you may be denying them the best treatment. However, you must not prescribe anything they say they are allergic to, unless you are confident they are not!

Family history

Ask about the cause, and age, of death of close relatives, especially parents and siblings. Practise drawing quick sketches of family trees (Fig. 21.2). Is there a specific family history pertinent to the suspected diagnosis?

186

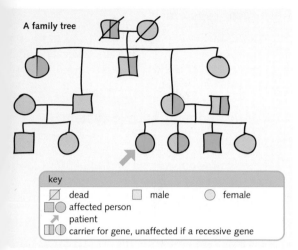

A family tree

key
- ⊠ dead   ▢ male   ○ female
- ▢○ affected person
- ↗ patient
- ▢◑ carrier for gene, unaffected if a recessive gene

Fig. 21.2 Example of Mendelian recessive inheritence depicted in a family tree. Arrow indicates the propositus, or individual who brought the pedigree to notice.

Social history

The purpose of this assessment is to see the patient in the context of their environment and gain some idea of how the illness affects this particular patient, what support the patient has and whether he or she can reduce any health risks.

It should include information about:

- Marital status.
- Children and other dependants.
- Occupational history (including previous occupations)—this is especially relevant regarding exposure to toxins, musculoskeletal disorders and psychiatry.
- Hobbies that may result in exposure to toxins or other risk.

- Accommodation—put yourself in the patient's position. Will he or she be able to cope at home? Are there stairs, lifts, bath, shower, etc.?
- Diet—is it adequate? High cholesterol? Vegetarian?
- Exercise—does he or she take any? Is it appropriate?

Is there any risk behaviour?

Consider the following:

- Ask about alcohol—record as units per day or week (Fig. 21.3).
- Ask about smoking—this is best described in terms of the number of 'pack-years', whereby 20 cigarettes smoked each day for 1 year is termed '1 pack year'. (Forty cigarettes a day for 3 years would equate to 'six pack years'.)
- Be tactful but thorough in asking about illicit or recreational drug use.
- Industrial toxins are important in claims for compensation (e.g. asbestos).
- A history of travel to certain regions of the world may be relevant.
- In addition to occupation or hobby, exposure to animals can be important.
- Sexual practice or orientation may be important for some conditions.

Review of symptoms (functional enquiry)

The purpose of this review is to go through the organ systems logically to ensure nothing is forgotten.

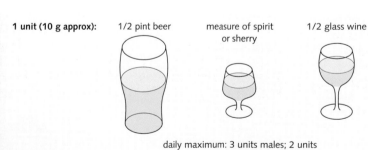

1 unit (10 g approx):   1/2 pint beer   measure of spirit or sherry   1/2 glass wine

daily maximum: 3 units males; 2 units females (or 21 and 14 per week)

- beer contains approximately 5% alcohol (i.e. 5 g/100 mL), i.e. 250 mL or 1/2 pint is 1 unit
- wine is usually about 12% alcohol: 750 mL standard bottle is 9 units, 1 unit per 1/2 glass
- spirits are often 40% alcohol: 25 mL measure is 1 unit

Fig. 21.3 Alcohol measures and recommended limits. Try to work out the units of alcohol for yourself. When working out measures, one unit of alcohol is rounded up to 10 g to simplify the calculations.

In addition, it often gives information into the cause or effect of the presenting complaint.

This can be very brief and some of the important questions to ask are listed. If the patient has any of these problems, clearly it is important to take a relevant extended history.

Gastrointestinal tract

Ask about:

- Abdominal pain.
- Indigestion.
- Nausea and vomiting.
- Heartburn.
- Dysphagia.
- Haematemesis and melaena.
- Jaundice.
- Abdominal swelling.
- Change of bowel habit.
- Diarrhoea.
- Rectal bleeding or pain.
- Weight loss.

(For a full discussion of these symptoms, refer to Part I.)

Cardiovascular system

Ask about chest pain:

- Related to exertion or posture?
- Relieved by rest?
- Are there any palpitations or postural syncopal attacks?
- Intermittent claudication is a sign of peripheral vascular disease. Ask patients how far they can walk before the pain comes on.
- Breathlessness can be a manifestation of cardiac disease.
- Orthopnoea refers to the patient being breathless when lying flat. This is due to increased hydrostatic pressure in the lungs consequent upon left ventricular dysfunction. It is usually measured in terms of the number of pillows required for sleeping. However, it is important to clarify why the patient uses several pillows—it may just be for a bad back!
- Paroxysmal nocturnal dyspnoea—the patient wakes up from the lying down position gasping for air for reasons similar to those for orthopnoea.

Respiratory system

Any chest pain? Is it 'pleuritic' or related to phases of respiration? Has there been any wheeze, cough or haemoptysis? If there is sputum, enquire about colour, nature and amount.

Endocrine and reproductive system

Has there been:

- Any polyuria or polydipsia (indicative of diabetes, hypercalcaemia)?
- Any heat or cold intolerance with mood change and/or weight change (suggestive of thyroid disease)?
- Any fatigue with pigmentation and dizzy spells (possibly Addison's disease)?
- Any erectile/fertility (male) or menstrual/fertility (female) problems?

Genitourinary tract

Is there any dysuria, nocturia, hesitancy, dribbling or incontinence, urethral discharge?

Central nervous system

Is there a history of specific symptoms, such as:

- Headache?
- Speech or visual disturbance?
- Dizzy spells?
- Fits or blackouts?
- Loss of power or sensation in any area?

Joints

Has there been pain or swelling in any joint, or any back pain?

Skin

Is there a skin rash, itchiness (pruritus) or lumps or bumps?

Try to formulate an impression or differential diagnosis based on the history before proceeding to examination. You may be able to anticipate abnormal physical signs.

Examination preliminaries

The main purpose of a general inspection is to determine how ill the patient is. Bear this in mind as you introduce yourself and take a history; if the patient is very ill, do not waste valuable time asking questions that can wait until later.

During the examination:

- Look at the patient's facial expression: is he or she comfortable, in obvious distress, looking furtive, receptive, hostile?
- Assess the patient's body posture and mobility, and his or her weight and size.
- Consider whether he or she is appropriately dressed and behaving appropriately in the circumstances.

Many diseases and conditions do not have a direct effect on the gut. However, always remember that the patient may be receiving medication for a pre-existing condition, and this may affect the dose of drug you are intending to give for his or her gastrointestinal (GI) condition (e.g. the patient may already be receiving enzyme-inducing drugs for another condition). Current medication may even be producing the gut symptoms (e.g. diarrhoea caused by antibiotic therapy).

> The purpose of the clinical examination is to find evidence in support of or against the differential diagnosis you are considering after taking the history. It should be thorough enough so as not to miss other possibilities that you had not considered, and to consider causes and effects of each putative diagnosis.

The following examination primer is orientated for GI disorders and is not comprehensive. You should read the relevant system in *Crash Course* for other disorders.

FACE

The face can be a mine of information. Some 'facies' are pathognomonic of certain conditions (e.g. dystrophia myotonica, Graves' disease and acromegaly), and have a peculiar habit of appearing in clinical examinations. Here, we concentrate on the facial signs of GI disease.

General inspection

Ask yourself the following questions:

- Are there any signs of mania or psychosis (possibly related to steroids, systemic lupus erythematosus, Wilson's disease, porphyria)?
- Is the patient agitated and not just anxious to see you (possible sign of hyperthyroidism, alcohol withdrawal)?
- Is the general appearance unkempt or neglected (e.g. due to alcohol or depression)?
- Is there excessive skin hair (hypertrichosis can occur with excess steroids, ciclosporin or minoxidil)?
- What is the skin's colour and its relevance (Fig. 22.1)?

Are there specific skin lesions suggestive of a particular disorder (Fig. 22.2), such as:

- Dermatitis herpetiformis (coeliac).
- Psoriasis (colitis, sometimes liver disease).
- Eczema (atopy).

Fig. 22.6 Signs relating to gastrointestinal pathology to be sought in the upper torso.

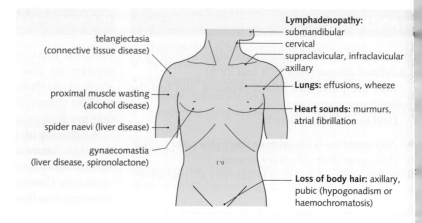

telangiectasia (connective tissue disease)

proximal muscle wasting (alcohol disease)

spider naevi (liver disease)

gynaecomastia (liver disease, spironolactone)

Lymphadenopathy:
submandibular
cervical
supraclavicular, infraclavicular
axillary
Lungs: effusions, wheeze
Heart sounds: murmurs, atrial fibrillation
Loss of body hair: axillary, pubic (hypogonadism or haemochromatosis)

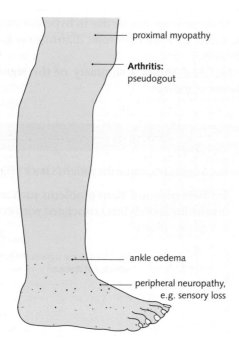

proximal myopathy

Arthritis:
pseudogout

ankle oedema

peripheral neuropathy, e.g. sensory loss

Fig. 22.7 Signs of gastrointestinal disease in the legs.

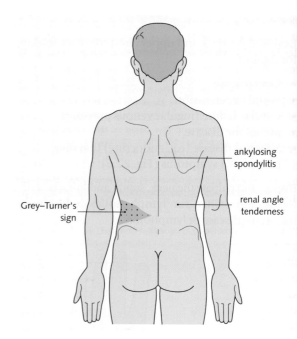

ankylosing spondylitis

Grey–Turner's sign

renal angle tenderness

Fig. 22.8 Examine the back for signs of intra-abdominal pathology.

- Tender renal angles from pyelonephritis may be an explanation for abdominal pain. Haemorrhagic pancreatitis may manifest as haematoma in the flanks or back (Grey–Turner's sign).

ABDOMINAL EXAMINATION

Warm your hands before you start or you may produce reflex guarding. Stand at the end of the bed and inspect the abdomen. Ask the patient to lift their head up from the pillow. This simple manoeuvre involves the abdominal wall muscles and can provide useful information: it may accentuate or reveal abdominal masses, organomegaly or asymmetry; and a patient with peritonitis will not be able to do it! Inspect for:

- Asymmetry.
- Lumps and bumps.
- Pulsation.
- Peristalsis.
- Scars.
- Distension.

Now move on to palpation. Position yourself at an appropriate level to the abdomen but maintain a steady posture. Adopting a kneeling position is often best, but make sure you check the floor surface first! During palpation it is helpful to form a visual map in your mind of normal intra-abdominal anatomy. Some abdominal organs may be just palpable in thin, normal subjects. Be systematic in your approach, palpating each contiguous area in turn.

Use superficial palpation initially to detect tenderness or guarding. Your hand should simply rest on the abdominal surface, and employ a gentle flexing action at the metacarpal-phalangeal joints. Follow with deep palpation, using a similar technique, to detect organomegaly and masses. Do not hurt the patient; watch their face! If you detect a mass, you need to be able to provide an accurate description. Note its position, size, shape, upper and lower borders, whether it is ballotable. Is it tender, hard, smooth or irregular? To determine whether it is pulsatile, lay your hand still for several seconds. Does it move with respiration?

Following systematic superficial and deep palpation of the abdomen, specifically seek evidence of hepatomegaly or splenomegaly. Begin palpation in the right iliac fossa, as both these organs can enlarge to this extent. Use the lateral border of your hand/forefinger and palpate in a parallel fashion, toward the right or left upper quadrant for the liver and spleen respectively. For each palpation, the patient should inspire and exhale as you press. You may feel the edge of the enlarged organ 'meet' your hand during inspiration. Now attempt to 'ballot' the kidneys. For each kidney in turn, slide one hand under the loin area while firmly pressing over the kidney with your other hand. The hand underneath should attempt to 'bounce' the kidney upward, while the other hand should remain still, and attempt to feel any abnormality.

Percussion is useful to confirm enlargement of the liver, spleen or distended bladder, if present. This is performed in the usual way and a dull note signifies a solid viscera or fluid collection beneath. Always percuss beyond both the upper and lower borders of the mass; remember that the liver can be 'pushed down' by hyperinflated lungs and appear enlarged, unless the upper border is determined by percussion. Percussion is also discriminatory if the abdomen is distended, to differentiate fluid (dull) from air (tympanitic).

You must know how to check for:

- Shifting dullness (dull percussion note becomes resonant when you roll the patient and gravity shifts the fluid).

- A fluid thrill (this can transmit 'tapping' from one side of the abdomen to the other).

Listen for bowel sounds and bruits. Accentuated auscultation (listening with the stethoscope over the solid structure while lightly scratching over the organ edge) can also be used to confirm liver or spleen enlargement.

Check inguinal, scrotal and umbilical hernial orifices, particularly in the scenario of intestinal obstruction.

Expected normal findings on examination of the abdomen are shown in Fig. 22.9.

The abnormal abdomen

Inspect the abdomen for scars—you need to be aware of their possible significance as, occasionally, the patient is not (Fig. 22.10). Any abnormality detected should be characterized carefully; establish whether an organ is involved and evaluate the nature of the mass. Does it move with respiration?

Masses or organomegaly in particular should be measured (cm) and commented on as in Fig. 22.11. Causes of common abdominal masses are listed in Fig. 22.12.

During superficial palpation for guarding and tenderness, be sure to look at the patient's face to check for reaction to pain. The purpose of the clinical examination is to find evidence in support of or against the differential diagnosis you are considering after taking the history. It should be thorough enough so as not to miss other possibilities that you had not considered, and to consider causes and effects of each putative diagnosis.

RECTAL EXAMINATION

This is a very important part of GI examination, but must be carried out properly or it is not worth doing. Clearly, there are sensitive issues of modesty and cultural code of which you need to be aware. Examination of a patient without consent may constitute an assault, and the more intimate

BROWN, Jane. 29/4/79

> 4. Name and date of birth on each side of clerking.

O/E   Looks well
       Overweight
       No evidence jaundice/anaemia/cyanosis
       No lymphadenopathy or goitre
       Clinically euthyroid
       P 80/minute + regular BP 120/62
       JVP normal
       HS I + II + 0
       Chest resonant + clear throughout

> 5. Record your initial observations – they are important. 'Alert & chatty' or 'Distressed & looks unwell' tell you a lot about the patient.

°L   °S

       No peripheral oedema
       No herniae
       PR + sigmoidoscopy to 15cm
       Normal mucosa
       'Pellet' stool

       Tender
       but not
       marked
       + no guarding

> 6. Always use diagrams to clarify your examination findings.

CNS   Grossly intact. GCS 15 PERLA
       Alert and responsive.

> 7. If there is no abnormality of the CNS, simply include a one-line summary.

Imp   △ Irritable bowel syndrome

Plan   Explanation, reassurance and advice
       Review in outpatients to reinforce
       + plan to discharge at 3 month followup
       Blood tests: FBC (to exclude anaemia),
       CRP/ESR (to look for evidence of infection
       or inflammation)
       Further investigation not indicated
       at this stage

> 8. Always include a management plan – even when you are still a student. It might not be right but you need to start training yourself to think like a doctor.

FOX 752

> 9. Sign your notes, including printed surname and bleep number.

Objectives

You should be able to:

- Understand the changes in routine haematology tests that occur in gastrointestinal disease
- Interpret the gut hormone profile
- Understand the significance of abnormalities of liver biochemistry
- Describe tests of pancreatic function
- Understand the breath tests utilized in the investigation of gastrointestinal disease
- Understand how upper gastrointestinal motility is assessed
- Interpret serological tests used in gastrointestinal disease
- Understand when to use and how to interpret tumour markers in the investigation of gastrointestinal disease
- Understand the factors that influence the choice of imaging modality used to investigate gastrointestinal disease

Investigations are used to confirm, reinforce or refute a differential diagnosis. You ought to be able to justify any test you order on clinical grounds. Brief notes follow to aid interpretation of tests in gastrointestinal (GI) disease.

ROUTINE HAEMATOLOGY

A full blood count (FBC) tends to be performed routinely on every patient and can provide vital information if interpreted correctly (Fig. 24.1).

A blood film can be very valuable if anaemia is present:

- Red cells can appear small (microcytosis), with variation of size (anisocytosis) and shape (poikilocytosis), in iron-deficiency anaemia. Red cells are also small in β-thalassaemia.
- Red cells are large (macrocytic) in vitamin B_{12} or folate deficiency and also in alcoholic liver disease.

Reticulocytes may be raised following recent blood loss and can account for a spurious macrocytosis on an automated FBC result. Target cells (ringed red blood cells) are common in liver disease. Be wary of a combined deficiency of vitamin B_{12}/folate and iron, resulting in both microcytes and macrocytes. This can appear as a normocytic anaemia.

A high platelet count (thrombocytosis) may be seen in cases of chronic blood loss or inflammatory disease.

Other haematological investigations can be helpful in GI disease:

- Vitamin B_{12}—if low, consider gastric or ileal resection, or disease (e.g. pernicious anaemia, Crohn's disease), blind loop syndrome, bacterial overgrowth, malabsorption. Disruption of liver architecture can lead to high levels (e.g. fibrolamellar hepatoma—rare) or hepatic abscess.
- Schilling test—replacing deficient intrinsic factor allows radiolabelled vitamin B_{12} to be absorbed (e.g. gastrectomy, pernicious anaemia: positive test), but has no effect if absorptive (ileal) mucosa is absent or diseased (e.g. ileal resection, Crohn's disease, tuberculosis: negative test) (Fig. 24.2).
- Folate can be low with any chronic debilitating state, malabsorption, excess alcohol and certain drugs (e.g. sulphonamides, colestyramine, anticonvulsants). It can be elevated in small intestinal bacterial overgrowth.

Routine biochemistry		
Parameter	**Level**	**GI significance**
Urea	Low High	Malabsorption or liver disease Slightly (up to 14 mmol/L): dehydration (nausea, vomiting, Addison's) Moderate (up to 20 mmol/L): profound dehydration, GI bleed (protein load) Severe (more than 20 mmol/L): renal failure, hepatorenal syndrome
Sodium (Na)	Low	Common in diarrhoea, vomiting, alcoholic liver disease, diuretics
Potassium (K)	Low High	Common in diarrhoea, vomiting, alcoholic liver disease, loop diuretics Possible renal failure, diuretics especially spironolactone
Calcium (Ca)	Low High	Correct for albumin, common in coeliac disease Associated with malignant disease, hyperparathyroidism
Magnesium (Mg)	Low	Commonly in malnutrition, malabsorption, alcoholic diseases
Creatinine	High	Renal failure (all causes)
Glucose	High	Hyperglycaemia can cause abdominal pain, dehydration and acidosis Acute and chronic pancreatitis can lead to high glucose in serum

Fig. 24.3 Routine biochemistry and its significance in gastrointestinal disease.

ENDOCRINE AND METABOLIC

Thyroid function

Thyroid disease does not usually cause GI problems, but may accentuate symptoms such as diarrhoea (hyperthyroidism) or constipation (hypothyroidism) from other causes. Hyperthyroidism needs to be excluded as a cause of weight loss (in children, it can cause weight gain!). Thyroid dysfunction can cause abnormal liver enzymes.

Catecholamine levels

A 24-hour urinary collection for free catecholamines (adrenaline (epinephrine), noradrenaline (norepinephrine) and dopamine) is used to diagnose catecholamine excess secondary to tumours of the adrenal medulla. These may present with GI symptoms of weight loss, nausea, vomiting and altered bowel habit. Associated features are flushing and cardiovascular dysfunction (arrhythmias and episodic hypertension). Note that some hospitals still measure urinary vanillylmandelic acid as a surrogate of catecholamine excess.

Cortisol

An absent or impaired cortisol response following administration of an analogue of adrenocorticotrophic hormone is useful to diagnose Addison's disease. This can present with nausea, vomiting, weight loss, diarrhoea or postural dizziness. Acute adrenal failure may present as severe abdominal pain, mimicking an acute abdomen.

Gut hormone profile

Serum gastrin

Serum gastrin is raised slightly in patients with *Helicobacter pylori* infection, peptic ulcer disease or in patients on long-term treatment with proton pump inhibitors. It is markedly raised in gastrinomas. These neuroendocrine tumours arise most commonly in the pancreas, but also in the mucosa of the duodenum or antrum. They present with peptic ulcers, diarrhoea and weight loss.

Urinary 5-hydroxyindole acetic acid

5-Hydroxyindole acetic acid (5-HIAA) is a breakdown product of 5-hydroxytryptamine (5-HT, serotonin) produced by argentaffin cells. Primary carcinoid tumours arise in the small intestine or rectum. The clinical syndrome of 5-HT excess only occurs when there are liver metastases, as 'first-pass' hepatic metabolism is avoided. It comprises abdominal pain and watery diarrhoea. Associated features are facial flushing and respiratory wheeze.

Vasoactive intestinal peptide

Vasoactive intestinal peptide is produced in excess by rare pancreatic tumours and causes severe watery diarrhoea.

Glucagon

Glucagon is produced in excess by alpha cell tumours of the pancreas, producing diabetes mellitus and a characteristic skin rash.

Somatostatinomas

Somatostatinomas produce diarrhoea and weight loss with diabetes mellitus.

Porphyrins

These are intermediate metabolites in the haem biosynthetic pathway. Enzyme absence or deficiency in the pathway results in their accumulation, leading to:

- Neuropsychiatric disorder.
- Hypertension.
- Photosensitive skin rashes.
- Abdominal pain.
- Hyponatraemia.

Excess porphobilinogen is found in urine. Red blood cell porphobilinogen deaminase and aminolaevulinic acid synthase, the most common enzyme deficiencies, can be measured (Fig. 24.4).

Nutrient elements

Iron

Serum iron is subject to too much fluctuation to be useful on its own. When compared with its binding capacity (total iron binding capacity), the percentage saturation of transferrin can be derived:

- Values below 20% are considered iron deficient.
- Values above 50% are probably iron overloaded.

(See Ch. 11.)

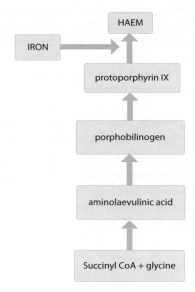

Fig. 24.4 Haem biosynthetic pathway.

Ferritin

Ferritin reflects body iron stores in adults and is a useful tool for investigating iron overload. However, as an acute-phase protein, it is elevated in any cause of inflammation. It can therefore be misleadingly normal or high in rheumatoid arthritis. It is also elevated in alcoholic hepatitis with which it may be difficult to differentiate from haemochromatosis.

Caeruloplasmin

A plasma protein that binds copper, caeruloplasmin is reduced in most cases of Wilson's disease, but this is not sufficient to make a diagnosis. Serum copper should also be elevated and 24-hour urinary copper excretion increased.

Zinc

Zinc is low in alcoholic liver disease; its deficiency can cause an enteropathy as well as skin rashes.

LIVER ENZYMES AND LIVER FUNCTION TESTS

Liver enzymes

Elevated liver enzymes in serum signify hepatic injury of some kind, but give no information about liver

Fig. 24.11 Method for assessing oesophageal pH: a nasogastric tube with a probe sensitive to hydrogen ions is placed 5 cm above the gastro-oesophageal junction. pH here should be greater than 4. Dips below this identify episodes of gastro-oesophageal acid reflux. This is represented by the waveforms shown in Fig. 24.12.

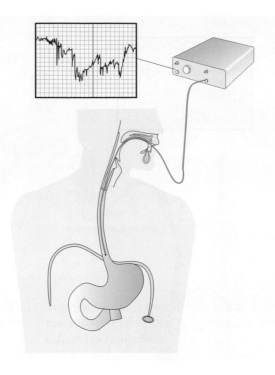

Fig. 24.12 Example of 24-hour pH recording from a patient with significant acid reflux. pH dipping below 4 indicates acid reflux from the stomach.

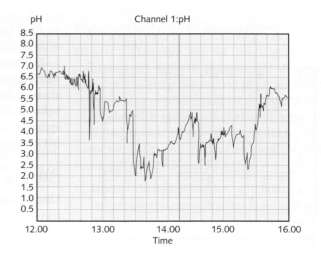

and enzyme-linked immunosorbent assay (ELISA) kits (Fig. 24.13). Their principal use is to screen for infection, tumours or immunoinflammatory disease when those conditions are suspected by the clinical presentation or the results of other tests.

These are useful confirmatory tests, but are much less useful and often confusing if used as screening tests. Here, they are classified according to their clinical implications in GI pathology.

Markers of autoimmune disease

Antibodies to various nuclear components are found in a number of diseases (Fig. 24.14), but also in up to 20% of the normal population.

More specific antibodies to double-stranded DNA are found in 50% of patients with systemic lupus erythematosus, and speckled pattern antinuclear factor in mixed connective tissue disease.

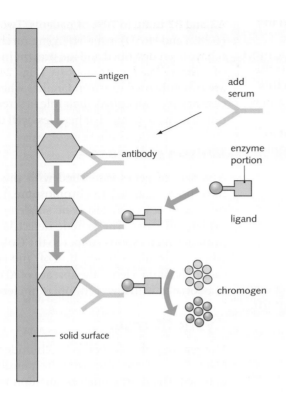

Fig. 24.13 The principles of enzyme-linked immunosorbent assay (ELISA). A solid surface is labelled with antigen (the solid phase). The patient's serum is added and if the specific antibody is present, it is held by the antigen and can be detected by a labelled antibody sandwich technique with a colouring agent.

Common autoantibodies		
Test	**Significance**	**Application**
Anti-mitochondrial Ab	PBC	When biliary enzymes raised
Anti-smooth muscle Ab	AICAH	When ALT raised
Anti-LKM Ab	AICAH	When ALT raised
Anti-nuclear Ab	CAH	When ALT raised
Anti-dsDNA Ab	SLE	Abnormal LFTs
Anti-gliadin Ab, Anti-endomysial antibodies and Anti-tissue transglutaminase Ab	Coeliac	In chronic diarrhoea/malabsorption
Anti-neutrophil cytoplasmic Ab	Ulcerative colitis	In blood diarrhoea

Fig. 24.14 Common autoantibodies and gastrointestinal disease. (Ab, antibody; AICAH, autoimmune chronic active hepatitis; ALT, alanine aminotransferase; dsDNA, double-stranded DNA; LFT, liver function test; LKM, liver–kidney microsomal (antibody); PBC, primary biliary cirrhosis; SLE, systemic lupus erythematosus.)

- Smooth muscle antibodies are found in 60% of cases of autoimmune chronic active hepatitis. Anti-liver–kidney microsomal antibodies are found in a subgroup of these patients with a more protracted course of disease.
- Gastric parietal cell antibodies are found in 90% of patients with pernicious anaemia.

- Rheumatoid factor (IgM class autoantibody against own IgG) is found in 70% of patients with rheumatoid-like arthritis and is the determining factor for seropositivity, which tends to run a more severe course.
- Anti-neutrophil cytoplasmic antibodies (ANCA) are found in a variety of connective tissue diseases, but the perinuclear variety (pANCA)

Multiple-choice questions (MCQs)

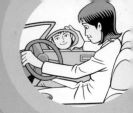

Indicate whether each answer is true or false.

1. **The following are true of pain arising from the oesophagus:**
   a. It is often precipitated by exertion
   b. It can occur in the absence of heartburn
   c. It can mimic the pain of a myocardial infarction
   d. It is never relieved by glyceryl trinitrate
   e. It is associated with *Helicobacter pylori*

2. **The following are true of the investigation of indigestion:**
   a. A microcytic anaemia would be unconcerning
   b. Positive *H. pylori* serology indicates current infection
   c. The onset of melaena would prompt urgent investigation
   d. A chest X-ray is diagnostically unhelpful
   e. The presence of a hiatus hernia is diagnostic of acid reflux

3. **The following statements are true:**
   a. Elevated tone of the lower oesophageal sphincter (LOS) contributes to acid reflux
   b. Smoking increases LOS tone
   c. Normal endoscopy excludes oesophageal reflux
   d. Pregnancy predisposes towards symptoms of reflux
   e. Conservative treatment is rarely effective in the management of acid reflux

4. **The following are true of Barrett's oesophagus:**
   a. Columnar epithelium is replaced by squamous epithelium
   b. It is a premalignant condition
   c. Endoscopic surveillance may be required
   d. The clinical features differ from reflux oesophagitis
   e. Severe dysplastic change is an ominous sign

5. **The following apply to a history of dysphagia:**
   a. Benign oesophageal stricture is often preceded by a history of heartburn
   b. If progressive, suggests globus hystericus
   c. The patient can accurately assess the level at which it occurs
   d. Associated regurgitation of food suggests a benign stricture
   e. Significant weight loss is suggestive of carcinoma

6. **In the investigation of dysphagia:**
   a. Barium swallow is preferable to endoscopy if there is a history of regurgitation
   b. A chest X-ray may demonstrate evidence of prior pulmonary infection
   c. Endoscopic ultrasound best assesses local spread of oesophageal carcinoma
   d. If a stricture is suspected, endoscopy is the most appropriate investigation
   e. A full blood count is rarely necessary

7. **The following are true of achalasia:**
   a. Endoscopy is a sensitive diagnostic test
   b. A history of regurgitation is common
   c. It oftens presents in childhood
   d. Retrosternal chest pain is a frequent symptom
   e. Histology shows a reduction of Auerbach plexus ganglia cells in the oesophageal wall

8. **In the context of acute abdominal pain:**
   a. An elevated amylase is always indicative of acute pancreatitis
   b. An electrocardiogram is an important investigation
   c. The presence of ascites may suggest Budd–Chiari syndrome
   d. Respiratory rate is a useful parameter to assess
   e. A patient with peritonitis will be restless with the pain

9. **The following are bad prognostic factors in acute pancreatitis:**
   a. High white cell count
   b. High calcium levels
   c. High blood urea
   d. High amylase levels
   e. Hypoxia—PO_2 <8

10. **The following are true of the investigation of acute abdominal pain:**
    a. Microscopic haematuria would support a diagnosis of renal colic
    b. The absence of subdiaphragmatic gas on a chest X-ray excludes perforation
    c. A high C-reactive protein can be found in Crohn's disease
    d. Biliary colic is supported by high levels of liver enzymes
    e. An abdominal ultrasound is unhelpful

11. **The following clinical features are associated with peptic ulcer disease:**
    a. A history of non-steroidal anti-inflammatory drug (NSAID) use
    b. Exacerbation of pain following eating
    c. The passage of fresh blood per rectum
    d. A palpable supraclavicular lymph node
    e. Radiation of pain to the back

12. The following are true of the investigation of chronic abdominal pain:

a. A normal amylase excludes chronic pancreatitis
b. A plain abdominal radiograph can be diagnostic
c. Thrombocytosis can indicate a chronic inflammatory process
d. Crohn's disease can present acutely with right iliac fossa pain
e. A macrocytic anaemia is found with chronic blood loss

13. The following are true of abdominal ascites:

a. Ascites with high protein content is found in the nephrotic syndrome
b. Absence of malignant cells on cytological examination excludes cancer
c. An echocardiogram may be indicated in its investigation
d. Ultrasonography is a sensitive diagnostic modality
e. Assessment of jugular venous pressure is important

14. For a patient with weight loss:

a. The patient's subjective assessment is usually accurate
b. Malignancy can cause weight loss through anorexia
c. Increased appetite may indicate hyperthyroidism
d. Hypocalcaemia may suggest malabsorption
e. Corticosteroid therapy may be a contributing factor

15. The following drugs are known to commonly cause vomiting:

a. Corticosteroids
b. Digoxin
c. Antibiotics (e.g. metronidazole)
d. NSAIDs
e. Morphine

16. The following metabolic conditions tend to produce vomiting:

a. Diabetic ketoacidosis
b. Hypoglycaemia
c. Hypercalcaemia
d. Hypocalcaemia
e. Uraemia

17. The following are true of upper gastrointestinal bleeding:

a. Haematemesis and melaena rarely occur together
b. The presence of a prosthetic heart valve influences management
c. A postural drop in blood pressure may indicate a significant bleed
d. The haemoglobin may be normal at the presentation of a large bleed
e. A history of preceding vomiting suggests peptic ulcer disease

18. In the investigation of upper gastrointestinal bleeding:

a. An elevated blood urea indicates chronic liver disease
b. A coagulopathy can be expected with peptic ulcer disease
c. A high leucocyte count can be seen in the context of a large bleed
d. Thrombocytopenia can be associated with bleeding oesophageal varices
e. Endoscopy is not always necessary

19. The following features dictate that a gastrointestinal bleed is 'high risk':

a. Age over 65 years
b. NSAIDs
c. Coexisting cardiac failure
d. Renal impairment
e. A low haemoglobin at presentation

20. The following drugs are well recognized to cause diarrhoea:

a. Codeine
b. Amoxicillin
c. Colchicine
d. Corticosteroids
e. Metronidazole

21. Blood-stained diarrhoea is associated with the following conditions:

a. Ulcerative colitis
b. Giardiasis
c. Radiation colitis
d. Irritable bowel syndrome
e. Thyrotoxicosis

22. The following are true of the investigation of diarrhoea:

a. Macrocytic anaemia suggests underlying inflammatory bowel disease
b. A 24-hour urine collection may be helpful
c. Bacterial cultures are frequently positive in diarrhoea of infective origin
d. Ferritin may be elevated in inflammatory bowel disease
e. An abdominal radiograph is frequently of diagnostic value

23. Steatorrhoea is associated with the following conditions:

a. Coeliac disease
b. Bacterial overgrowth
c. Chronic pancreatitis
d. Ileal tuberculosis
e. Whipple's disease

24. The following organisms are frequently implicated in infective diarrhoea:

a. Rotavirus
b. Cytomegalovirus
c. *Salmonella* sp.
d. *Staphylococcus aureus*
e. Cryptosporidiosis

25. **The following biochemical derangements can be associated with diarrhoea:**
   a. Elevated blood urea
   b. Hyperkalaemia
   c. Hypomagnesaemia
   d. Hypercalcaemia
   e. Hyperglycaemia

26. **In the context of rectal bleeding:**
   a. Haemorrhoids produce dark red 'venous' bleeding
   b. Red blood mixed with stool is associated with low rectal lesions
   c. Pain on defecation is a feature of anal fissure
   d. Tenderness in the left iliac fossa suggests angiodysplasia
   e. Anaemia can usually be attributed to the blood loss

27. **The following are true of the investigation of rectal bleeding:**
   a. The majority of conditions can be diagnosed clinically with proctoscopy and sigmoidoscopy
   b. Angiography is only indicated if there is active bleeding at the time
   c. Rigid sigmoidoscopy can identify lesions up to 35 cm from the anal margin
   d. Anal fissure is frequently seen during proctoscopy
   e. The presence of haemorrhoids on proctoscopy makes more invasive investigation unnecessary

28. **In the patient with anaemia:**
   a. Conjunctival pallor is a sensitive correlate to the haemoglobin concentration
   b. Further tests are dependent on the full blood count parameters
   c. Gastroscopy should be undertaken in all cases of iron-deficient anaemia in the absence of an alternative explanation
   d. The presence of a duodenal ulcer is an adequate explanation for iron-deficiency anaemia
   e. Coeliac disease is an uncommon cause of malabsorption with anaemia in this country

29. **The following are true of macrocytic anaemia:**
   a. Methotrexate and anticonvulsant drugs can lead to vitamin B_{12} deficiency
   b. A reticulocytosis can result in a spurious macrocytosis
   c. Caecal carcinoma is a common cause in the elderly
   d. A Schilling test may be indicated if folate levels are low
   e. Hypothyroidism is a recognized cause

30. **The following are true of iron deficiency:**
   a. It is confirmed by a low serum iron *and* a low iron-binding capacity
   b. Non-steroidal anti-inflammatory drugs are commonly implicated
   c. It can result from heavy menstruation
   d. It can be a manifestation of coeliac disease
   e. Oval macrocytes are seen on a peripheral blood film

31. **The following statements regarding jaundice are true:**
   a. It is only detectable clinically when the serum bilirubin level exceeds 80 µmol/L
   b. A rapid onset suggests autoimmune disease
   c. A palpable gall bladder suggests gallstones as the cause
   d. Abdominal ultrasound is the key investigation
   e. The level of bilirubin reflects hepatic synthetic function

32. **The following drugs are known to cause jaundice:**
   a. Flucloxacillin
   b. Paracetamol
   c. Aspirin
   d. Gentamicin
   e. Antituberculous drugs

33. **The following clinical findings can be associated with jaundice:**
   a. Lymphadenopathy
   b. Ascites
   c. Extrapyramidal neurological signs
   d. Palmar erythema
   e. Peripheral oedema

34. **Regarding liver biochemistry:**
   a. Alanine aminotransferase (ALT) is a good reflection of liver function
   b. Elevated gamma-glutamyl transferase (GGT) can also reflect bony metastases or Paget's disease
   c. GGT is an enzyme easily 'induced' by drugs or alcohol
   d. Elevated ALT and bilirubin suggests liver metastases
   e. T-cell lymphomas can derange liver enzymes

35. **The following conditions cause clubbing of the nails:**
   a. Coeliac disease
   b. Caecal carcinoma
   c. Crohn's disease
   d. Chronic pancreatitis
   e. Cirrhosis

36. **The following clinical signs are correctly matched to the underlying condition:**
   a. Grey–Turner's sign and acute pancreatitis
   b. Proximal myopathy and alcoholism
   c. Splenomegaly and cirrhosis
   d. Cullen's sign and Crohn's disease
   e. Pyoderma gangrenosum and ulcerative colitis

37. **The following haematological findings are correctly matched to the disorder:**
   a. Thrombocytosis and portal hypertension
   b. Neutrophilia and colonic inflammation
   c. Macrocytosis and iron deficiency
   d. Thrombocytosis and inflammatory disease
   e. Leucopenia and viral hepatitis

38. **The following conditions typically cause pain in the right iliac fossa:**
    a. Ectopic pregnancy
    b. Biliary colic
    c. Appendicitis
    d. Diverticulitis
    e. Crohn's disease

39. **The following are recognized causes of a right iliac fossa mass:**
    a. Ileocaecal tuberculosis
    b. Appendicitis
    c. Caecal carcinoma
    d. Coeliac disease
    e. Ectopic pregnancy

40. **The following skin lesions can be associated with disease of the gastrointestinal tract:**
    a. Dermatitis herpetiformis
    b. Psoriasis
    c. Eczema
    d. Spider naevi
    e. Xanthelasmata

41. **The following investigations are usually indicated following an acute upper gastrointestinal bleed:**
    a. Endoscopy
    b. Endoscopic retrograde cholangiopancreatography
    c. Laparoscopy
    d. Labelled red blood cell scan
    e. Barium meal

42. **The following statements regarding reflux oesophagitis are true:**
    a. It may manifest with nocturnal coughing
    b. Iron-deficiency anaemia can result
    c. The condition is more common in asthmatics
    d. Lying flat relieves symptoms
    e. It can mimic the pain of cardiac ischaemia

43. **The following drugs may exacerbate symptoms of dyspepsia/reflux:**
    a. Tricyclic antidepressants
    b. Domperidone
    c. Non-steroidal anti-inflammatory drugs
    d. Caffeine
    e. Proton pump inhibitors

44. **The following are potential complications of reflux oesophagitis:**
    a. Upper gastrointestinal bleeding
    b. Barrett's oesophagus
    c. Acute pancreatitis
    d. Benign oesophageal stricture
    e. Peptic ulceration

45. **The following are true of Barrett's oesophagus:**
    a. The majority of people with prolonged reflux will develop Barrett's
    b. Metaplastic change is from columnar to squamous epithelium
    c. Histological change correlates poorly with symptomatology
    d. Proton pump inhibitor therapy may allow return of normal epithelium
    e. Long-term endoscopic surveillance is often indicated

46. **The following are true of benign oesophageal strictures:**
    a. Weight loss can be marked
    b. Symptoms can mimic those of malignant strictures
    c. Symptoms of acid reflux often worsen as the condition progresses
    d. Endoscopic ultrasound may be necessary to exclude malignant infiltration
    e. A history of radiotherapy to the mediastinum may be pertinent

47. **In the context of oesophageal carcinoma:**
    a. Retrosternal chest pain is the commonest presenting feature
    b. Pernicious anaemia is associated
    c. The majority are squamous cell carcinomas
    d. Radiotherapy is often curative
    e. An elevated ALT and GGT may be seen

48. **Regarding the stomach:**
    a. The fundus extends to form the pylorus
    b. The antrum secretes gastrin from G cells
    c. An acidic pH is required to activate enzymes
    d. It is a major site of absorption of glucose and amino acids
    e. Chief cells secrete pepsinogen

49. **The following are true of *Helicobacter pylori*:**
    a. It is noted for its ability to produce the enzyme urease
    b. Asymptomatic infection is uncommon
    c. Increasing prevalence is seen with advancing age
    d. It is a Gram-negative bacterium
    e. Peptic ulceration is the only manifestation of infection

50. **Regarding diagnostic tests for *H. pylori*:**
    a. Culture of the organism is a rapid and sensitive method of detection
    b. A serological antibody test indicates current infection
    c. Oesophagogastroduodenoscopy may demonstrate a blotchy mucosal appearance
    d. A normal full blood count makes infection unlikely
    e. The urease breath test involves inhalation of radiolabelled urea

51. **The following are true of gastric ulcers:**
    a. They occur more commonly in the elderly
    b. They occur more commonly than duodenal ulceration
    c. Retrosternal pain is common
    d. Eating may precipitate pain
    e. May be painless

52. Complications of gastric ulceration include:

a. Gastric outflow obstruction
b. Iron-deficiency anaemia
c. Peritonitis
d. Pancreatitis
e. Dysphagia

53. In the context of duodenal ulceration:

a. Iron-deficiency anaemia is common
b. Association with *H. pylori* is unusual
c. The patient's blood group may be relevant
d. An acute gastrointestinal bleed may be the first manifestation
e. Recurrent disease is typical

54. The following investigations are indicated in the presence of gastric carcinoma:

a. Chest X-ray
b. Abdominal X-ray
c. Liver biochemistry
d. Renal ultrasound
e. Serum calcium

55. The following are recognized complications following gastrectomy:

a. Vitamin D deficiency
b. Bacterial overgrowth
c. Constipation
d. Diabetes mellitus
e. Anaemia

56. The following may be manifestations of small intestinal disease:

a. Steatorrhoea
b. Constipation
c. Weight loss
d. Osteomalacia
e. Abdominal pain

57. Regarding coeliac disease:

a. It is commonly seen in black Africans
b. Hypersplenism is associated
c. Intestinal lymphoma is associated
d. There are documented human leukocyte antigen (HLA) associations
e. A dimorphic blood picture may be seen

58. The following are recognized complications of coeliac disease:

a. T-cell lymphoma
b. Peripheral oedema
c. Macrocytic anaemia
d. Microcytic anaemia
e. Eczema

59. The following abnormalities can be seen in Crohn's disease:

a. Normocytic anaemia
b. Low albumin
c. Low platelet count
d. High C-reactive protein
e. High serum calcium

60. The following are systemic manifestations of Crohn's disease:

a. Uveitis
b. Myocarditis
c. Seropositive arthritis
d. Osteopenia
e. Pyoderma gangrenosum

61. The following statements are true of GI manifestations of Crohn's disease:

a. Oral ulceration is common
b. Transmural inflammation with non-caseating granulomas is seen
c. The rectum is commonly involved
d. Inflammation tends to be contiguous along the bowel
e. Duodenal ulceration can occur

62. The following are true of Crohn's disease:

a. Corticosteroids improve the overall prognosis of the condition
b. Secondary amyloidosis can develop
c. A small proportion of patients require surgical intervention
d. Immunosuppression can be effective, even in severe disease
e. Anaerobic infections are common in perianal disease

63. The following features are seen in the carcinoid syndrome:

a. Abdominal pain
b. Constipation
c. Bronchoconstriction
d. Pulmonary stenosis
e. Peripheral neuropathy

64. The following are clinical features of bacterial overgrowth:

a. Peptic ulceration
b. Steatorrhoea
c. Vitamin B_{12} deficiency
d. Gastrointestinal bleeding
e. Weight loss

65. The following conditions are matched correctly to the type of organism responsible:

a. Giardiasis—anaerobe
b. Cholera—Gram-negative bacillus
c. Tuberculosis—protozoan
d. Yersinia—Gram-negative bacterium
e. Tropical sprue—unknown

66. Regarding the large intestine:

a. Its main role is the absorption of water and electrolytes
b. Absorption takes place predominantly in the ascending colon
c. The ascending colon is predominantly supplied by the inferior mesenteric artery
d. The ileocaecal valve heralds the end of the large intestine
e. The transverse colon is supplied solely by the superior mesenteric artery

67. The following statements regarding irritable bowel syndrome are true:

a. Abdominal pain with weight loss are typical features
b. Left iliac fossa pain relieved by defecation is common
c. Imaging of the large bowel is often diagnostically helpful
d. Increased fibre intake is universally helpful in symptom control
e. Psychological stress may be a precipitant

68. The following drugs commonly cause constipation:

a. Tricyclic antidepressants
b. Selective serotonin reuptake inhibitor antidepressants
c. Iron sulphate
d. Codeine phosphate
e. Thyroxine

69. The following statements are true of colitis:

a. Granulomas are present in collagenous colitis
b. Rectal sparing is characteristic of Crohn's colitis
c. Caseating granulomas in the terminal ileum are diagnostic of Crohn's disease
d. Colitis in a smoker is more likely to be Crohn's than ulcerative colitis
e. Pain is a characteristic feature of cytomegalovirus colitis

70. The following are true of ulcerative colitis:

a. It commonly presents with pain in the right iliac fossa
b. It can be associated with ankylosing spondylitis
c. It is a risk factor for toxic dilatation of the colon
d. The appearance of abdominal tenderness is an ominous sign
e. It often causes ischiorectal abscesses

71. The following are extra-intestinal features of ulcerative colitis:

a. Pyoderma gangrenosum
b. Renal calculi
c. Sclerosing cholangitis
d. Episcleritis
e. Mononeuritis multiplex

72. The following are true of ulcerative colitis:

a. Pseudopolyps can be seen macroscopically
b. Crypt abscesses and goblet cell depletion are typical
c. Long-standing colitis can lead to loss of haustra with fibrosis
d. Perinuclear anti-neutrophil cytoplasmic antibodies (pANCA) are often detected
e. The small intestine is never affected

73. The following features are indicative of severity in ulcerative colitis:

a. Fever
b. Vomiting
c. Tachycardia

d. Hypoalbuminaemia
e. Anaemia

74. The following are true of colon polyps and colon cancer:

a. The larger the polyp, the greater the risk of cancer
b. Malignant polyps can be successfully treated by colonoscopy and polypectomy alone
c. Hyperplastic polyps have a higher malignant potential than villous polyps
d. Polyps are common in the ascending colon
e. Colonic polyps are often recurrent

75. The following statements are true of colonic carcinoma:

a. Altered bowel habit is seen in greater than half of all patients
b. Rectal bleeding is common with right-sided lesions
c. Iron-deficiency anaemia is common with right-sided lesions
d. Jaundice can occur
e. It may present as an 'acute abdomen'

76. The following statements are true of bacterial infection of the colon:

a. It is a common cause of diarrhoea
b. Sigmoidoscopy is usually necessary
c. Leucocytosis may be seen
d. Anaemia is common
e. Antidiarrhoeal agents should be avoided

77. The following statements are true:

a. Amoebiasis can result in bloody diarrhoea
b. Cryptosporidiosis tends to be self-limiting in healthy individuals
c. Schistosomiasis can cause a localized granulomatous reaction in the colon
d. *Clostridium difficile* infection often follows treatment with narrow-spectrum antibiotics
e. Oral vancomycin can be used to treat *C. difficile*

78. The following are recognized functions of the liver:

a. Synthesis of all the coagulation factors
b. Iron storage
c. Excretion of bilirubin
d. Synthesis of insulin
e. Synthesis of albumin

79. With regard to hepatitis A virus (HAV) infection:

a. Prodromal symptoms can mimic viral gastroenteritis
b. Craving for nicotine is said to be enhanced in those who smoke
c. Splenomegaly is common in the icteric phase
d. Elevation of anti-HAV IgG implies acute infection
e. Myocarditis is a potential complication

80. The following statements regarding hepatitis B are correct:

a. Symptomless infected carrier rate can be up to 20% in some parts of the world
b. The average incubation period is 14–21 days

c. A polyarthritis can be a feature of acute infection
d. Up to 90% of acute infections resolve without sequelae
e. Carrier rate is much higher following vertical transmission

81. **The following statements regarding hepatitis B (HB) are true:**
    a. HBsAg (surface antigen) is the first serological marker to appear
    b. HBeAg ('e' antigen) reflects viral replication and high infectivity
    c. Anti-HBe antibodies appear late (>3 months)
    d. Anti-HBs antibodies confer lifelong immunity
    e. Transaminase levels peak at around the same time as HBeAg levels

82. **With regard to hepatitis C:**
    a. Routine screening of blood products for the virus has been available since 1978
    b. Clinical jaundice appears in the majority of patients
    c. Synthetic function is usually preserved
    d. Viral RNA can be detected by polymerase chain reaction (PCR)
    e. Approximately two-thirds of patients will progress to cirrhosis

83. **The following statements are true of infections involving the liver:**
    a. Atypical lymphocytes can be seen in the blood with infectious mononucleosis
    b. Hepatitis due to Epstein–Barr virus carries a poor prognosis
    c. Cytomegalovirus infection occurs predominantly in the immunocompromised
    d. Leptospirosis can be associated with renal failure
    e. Toxoplasmosis can cause a febrile illness with lymphadenopathy

84. **Haemochromatosis:**
    a. Is a genetic defect resulting in copper overload in the liver
    b. Is a risk factor for the development of hepatoma
    c. Has an equal sex incidence but presents earlier in males than females
    d. Can result in low blood glucose levels
    e. Can cause hypogonadism in the absence of cirrhosis

85. **With regard to primary sclerosing cholangitis:**
    a. It occurs predominantly in middle-aged females
    b. It is a major risk factor for cholangiocarcinoma
    c. It occurs in 50% of patients with ulcerative colitis
    d. Ursodeoxycholic acid may be of some benefit
    e. It may require insertion of an endoprosthesis for its treatment

86. **The following statements are true:**
    a. Kayser–Fleischer rings are seen in Wilson's disease
    b. Serum copper is grossly elevated (×10) in Wilson's disease

c. Upper lobe emphysema is seen in homozygotes with alpha-1-antitrypsin deficiency
d. In alpha-1-antitrypsin deficiency, prognosis depends on genotype
e. Splenomegaly can be seen in cystic fibrosis

87. **The following are recognized extra-pulmonary features of cystic fibrosis:**
    a. Diabetes insipidus
    b. Impotence
    c. Malabsorption
    d. Small bowel obstruction
    e. Cirrhosis

88. **With regard to primary biliary cirrhosis:**
    a. It predominantly affects women, with a ratio of 10:1
    b. Itching is a prominent feature, and often precedes jaundice
    c. Xanthomas are seen
    d. Vitamin D deficiency is common
    e. Membranous glomerulonephritis is associated

89. **The following statements regarding alcoholic liver disease are true:**
    a. The majority of people dependent on alcohol will develop liver disease
    b. Fatty change is reversible with abstinence from alcohol
    c. Mallory bodies are characteristic of alcohol damage
    d. Seventy-five per cent of liver cirrhosis is due to alcohol
    e. Macrocytosis may be seen

90. **The following are recognized stigmata of chronic liver disease:**
    a. Leuconychia
    b. Koilonychia
    c. Jaundice
    d. Palmar erythema
    e. Cyanosis

91. **The following features are used to assess functional capacity of the liver:**
    a. Serum bilirubin levels
    b. Serum albumin
    c. Serum glucose
    d. Encephalopathy
    e. Spider naevi

92. **The following are true of tumours of the liver:**
    a. Metastases are the commonest tumours seen in the liver
    b. Cirrhosis is a risk for hepatocellular carcinoma, whatever the cause
    c. Hepatocellular carcinomas are particularly sensitive to chemotherapy
    d. Liver ultrasound will detect the majority of liver tumours
    e. Haemangiomas are the commonest benign liver tumour

93. The following statements are true of paracetamol toxicity:

a. Glutathione depletion is a key biochemical feature
b. Patients with pre-existing liver impairment are at greater risk of hepatic damage
c. A prolonged prothrombin time correlates accurately with hepatic damage
d. An elevated creatinine is a poor prognostic feature
e. Metabolic alkalosis is seen

94. The following statements are true:

a. Unconjugated bilirubin is water soluble
b. Enterohepatic circulation of bilirubin occurs via the hepatic vein
c. The majority of patients with gallstones will require a cholecystectomy at some stage
d. The majority of gallstones are radio-opaque
e. Patients with terminal ileal disease are at risk of developing gallstones

95. The following are potential complications of gallstone disease:

a. Acute pancreatitis
b. Pancreatic carcinoma
c. Ascending cholangitis
d. Primary biliary cirrhosis
e. Empyema of the gall bladder

96. The following are true of infections involving the biliary tract:

a. Bile within the biliary tree is usually sterile
b. Septicaemic shock with Gram-negative organisms can occur
c. A 'cholestatic' picture may be seen biochemically
d. Blood cultures are rarely positive
e. Endoscopic retrograde cholangiopancreatography is a risk factor for cholangitis

97. The following are recognized clinical features of acute pancreatitis:

a. Hypovolaemic shock
b. Haematemesis
c. Upper abdominal pain
d. Vomiting
e. Hypoxia

98. The following are recognized causes of acute pancreatitis:

a. Hypocalcaemia
b. Hyperglycaemia
c. Corticosteroid therapy
d. Alcohol excess
e. Snake bite

99. The following are potential complications of acute pancreatitis:

a. Septicaemia
b. Hyperglycaemia
c. Disseminated intravascular coagulation
d. Ileus
e. Acute renal failure

100. The following statements are true:

a. Serum amylase is rarely normal in chronic pancreatitis
b. Endoscopic retrograde cholangiopancreatography may be useful in the diagnosis of chronic pancreatitis
c. Pseudocysts are an uncommon complication of acute pancreatitis
d. Thrombophlebitis migrans is associated with pancreatic carcinoma
e. Ascites occurs early in the course of pancreatic carcinoma

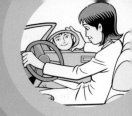

1. A 46-year-old woman presents with painless jaundice and pruritis. Alkaline phosphatase and gamma-glutamyl transferase are three to five times the upper limit of normal. Transaminases are normal. What would your initial choice of investigations be? Why is a history of respiratory tract infection, for which she received treatment, of relevance?

2. A 22-year-old female presents with acute abdominal pain. She is tachycardic and hypotensive. She has marked tenderness in the right iliac fossa with signs of localized peritonitis. List five possible diagnoses and suggest one key investigation that could confirm each.

3. A man aged 55 years is found to have a microcytic hypochromic anaemia on a routine full blood count. How would you confirm iron deficiency? An endoscopy reveals a duodenal ulcer. What would you do next?

4. A 38-year-old man presents with bloody diarrhoea with negative stool cultures and raised inflammatory markers. Describe five features that may help differentiate Crohn's disease from ulcerative colitis.

5. A 52-year-old man presents with severe upper abdominal pain and vomiting. Serum amylase is 3500. List the parameters that have prognostic significance and outline your initial management of the patient.

6. A 28-year-old man presents with diarrhoea. His brother is known to carry HLA-B27. What diagnostic possibilities should be considered for this patient and why?

7. A man aged 34 years presents with several weeks of diarrhoea and associated weight loss of 10 kg, despite a normal appetite. You suspect malabsorption. What biochemical and haematological tests would be relevant. List some causes of malabsorption and, given the history, name other conditions that could be easily excluded.

8. A 67-year-old man presented 3 months ago with obstructive jaundice. A diagnosis of carcinoma in the head of the pancreas was made and the obstruction was relieved by endoscopic insertion of a biliary stent. He now presents with jaundice, rigors, pyrexia and pain in the right upper quadrant. What is the most likely explanation, and how would you investigate and treat him? What might you expect to find on blood cultures?

9. A 52-year-old woman presents with a history that is strongly suggestive of peptic ulcer disease. What diagnostic options do you have in establishing her *Helicobacter pylori* status? She is confirmed *H. pylori* positive. Give an example of an eradication regimen that may be used. Why might a patient be advised to avoid alcohol while taking this course?

10. A young woman attends A&E after taking 30 paracetamol tablets earlier that day. Which other pieces of information are particularly relevant? How would you decide whether or not to administer *N*-acetylcysteine? What are the three main parameters that have prognostic significance?

11. A 17-year-old male is referred with a bilirubin of 60, alanine aminotransferase (ALT) normal, alkaline phosphatase slightly elevated and gamma-glutamyl transferase (GGT) normal. What is the most likely diagnosis and what is the mechanism of the hyperbilirubinaemia in this condition? Why is the alkaline phosphatase raised? List other situations in which an elevated alkaline phosphatase reflects a non-hepatological source.

12. A woman aged 70 years is found to have a macrocytic anaemia. Serum vitamin B_{12} levels are found to be low. She has a good diet. What tests could you perform to establish the aetiology of her vitamin B_{12} deficiency? What other causes of a macrocytic anaemia can you list?

13. A patient known to have hepatic cirrhosis is brought to A&E. He has become confused and disorientated over the last 2 days. He has a coarse flap with outstretched hands, sweet smelling breath and, shortly after admission, has a seizure lasting 1 minute. What is the diagnosis and what precipitants are commonly implicated in an acute onset such as this? Which four other parameters encompass the 'modified Child classification of cirrhosis'.

14. A man aged 32 years with recently diagnosed ulcerative colitis is admitted from the clinic. He has

been unwell for several days with profuse bloody diarrhoea, and feeling hot and shivery. List the clinical and laboratory features that would indicate severity in an exacerbation of ulcerative colitis such as this (up to eight). Which particular symptom would concern you? How would you explain the 'hot and shivery' symptoms? Outline your initial management of this patient.

15. A man aged 46 years is found to have an elevated alanine aminotransferase (ALT) and alkaline phosphatase and is subsequently investigated. Serum ferritin is found to be grossly elevated at 1200 and a presumptive diagnosis of haemochromatosis is made. How would you make a definitive diagnosis? Under what circumstances can an elevated ferritin be misleading? List the other manifestations of haemochromatosis according to the site affected.

Extended matching questions (EMQs)

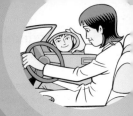

1. THEME: Haematemesis and melaena

A. Gastric ulceration
B. Oesophageal varices
C. Mallory–Weiss tear
D. Gastric carcinoma
E. Non-steroidal anti-inflammatory drug (NSAID)-associated peptic ulcer
F. Acute gastritis
G. Severe haemophilia
H. Atrophic gastritis
I. Duodenal ulceration

The patients below have all presented with evidence of upper gastrointestinal bleeding. Select the most appropriate diagnosis from the above list.

1. A 57-year-old lady presents to A&E with a 2-day history of tarry black stools but no abdominal pain. She has a history of rheumatoid arthritis for 10 years but has not needed immunosuppressive therapy. She looks pale, has no signs of chronic liver disease, abdominal examination is unremarkable and melaena is confirmed on rectal examination. ☐

2. A patient known to have alcoholic cirrhosis is brought in as an emergency after vomiting large amounts of fresh red blood and subsequently collapsing in the street. On examination, he is peripherally cold and clammy, hypotensive and tachycardic. There are signs of chronic liver disease evident. ☐

3. A young man of 19 years presents to A&E after noticing blood in his vomit. He had consumed excess alcohol that night and was vomiting repeatedly. He says he noticed the streaks of red blood on the last two episodes of vomiting. There are no abnormal examination findings and full blood count (FBC) and urea and electrolytes (U&E) are normal. ☐

4. A 70-year-old man presents to his GP with a 1-week history of tarry black stools. On questioning, he had been experiencing upper abdominal pain for some weeks. He was unsure how much weight he had lost, but his trousers had become very loose. Full blood count revealed a haemoglobin (Hb) 9.4 g/dL, mean cell volume (MCV) 76, platelets (Plt) 540, white cell count (WCC) 9.9. ☐

5. A 45-year-old man visits his GP with an intermittent history of epigastric pain. This seems to be relieved by food or antacids. He points to a specific site in his epigastrium where the pain is experienced. *Helicobacter pylori* serology is positive. ☐

2. THEME: Diarrhoea

A. Crohn's disease
B. Coeliac disease
C. Pseudomembranous colitis
D. Giardiasis
E. Colonic carcinoma
F. *Campylobacter* infection
G. Ulcerative colitis
H. Thyrotoxicosis
I. Appendicitis

The following patients all give a history of diarrhoea. Select the most likely diagnosis from the above list.

1. A 75-year-old Irish lady has had diarrhoea for a few months. This has been associated with 1 stone weight loss despite a normal appetite. On examination, she is pale and has a normal pulse rate. Iron-deficiency anaemia is found on blood tests and lower gastrointestinal investigations are normal. ☐

2. A 27-year-old man returns from a trip to Borneo. He has had watery diarrhoea for 10 days and has lost several kilograms in weight. Initial stool examination is negative but a repeat specimen is requested. There have been no previous episodes. ☐

3. A young woman has had diarrhoea for 1 week. There is no abdominal pain or blood. Her weight is stable. Past history only comprises treatment for a skin infection 2 weeks ago. Standard stool culture is negative. ☐

4. A man of 34 years presents to his GP with a 6-week history of diarrhoea associated with intermittent right iliac fossa pain. There is mucus but no blood on rectal examination. Blood tests demonstrate a normochromic normocytic anaemia with elevated C-reactive protein at 76. ☐

5. A woman of 62 years has experienced diarrhoea for several weeks and has visibly lost weight, despite a healthy appetite. She is very anxious about her change in bowel habit. She tells you that her father died of 'a stomach tumour'. On examination, she has a normal blood pressure but her pulse is irregular. There are no palpable abdominal masses and she declines rectal examination. ☐

3. THEME: Acute abdominal pain

A. Peptic ulceration
B. Biliary colic

7. THEME: Abnormal liver biochemistry

A. Hepatic metastases
B. Hepatitis C infection
C. Primary biliary cirrhosis
D. Drug-induced hepatitis
E. Congestive cardiac failure
F. Primary amyloidosis
G. Haemochromatosis
H. Hepatitis A infection
I. Constrictive pericarditis

The following patients have all been found to have abnormal liver biochemistry. Attempt to identify the most likely diagnosis from the list provided.

1. A man aged 72 years is found to have an alkaline phosphatase of 980, a GGT of 645 and an ALT of 78. Bilirubin and albumin are normal. He has peripheral oedema but no ascites and there is a resting tachycardia with an audible third heart sound. ☐

2. A man in his 20s presents to A&E with nausea and vomiting. He also has a dull headache and a temperature of 37.8 °C. On examination he has a 4-cm liver edge, a spleen tip is palpable and he is clearly jaundiced. Alkaline phosphatase 450, GGT 100, ALT 800, bilirubin 50. He is seen 4 weeks later and there has been complete clinical and biochemical resolution. ☐

3. A man aged 65 years is referred by the cardiologist for investigation of abnormal liver biochemistry. Alkaline phosphatase 1200, GGT 550, ALT 89, bilirubin 39, albumin 21. He is being treated for cardiac failure of unknown aetiology (coronary angiography normal). He has peripheral oedema but a normal pulse rate, blood pressure, jugular venous pressure (JVP) and heart sounds. Proteinuria ++ is found on dipstick. There is evidence of hepatomegaly on clinical examination. ☐

4. A woman aged 55 years is found to have abnormal liver biochemistry following investigation of a normocytic anaemia. Alkaline phosphatase 670, GGT 368, ALT and bilirubin normal. Albumin low at 29 and adjusted calcium 2.70. Clinical history is unrevealing. One week later, she fractures her right humerus following a fall in a shopping centre. ☐

5. A man aged 47 years is referred for investigation of the following abnormalities. Alkaline phosphatase 400, GGT 90, ALT 107, bilirubin 20, albumin 30. He gives a history of joint stiffness and loss of libido. On examination, he has a healthy complexion, but evidence of hepatomegaly. There is no active joint inflammation and glucose is found on urine dipstick. ☐

C. Carcinoma of the head of the pancreas
D. Alcoholic liver disease
E. Sclerosing cholangitis
F. Intrahepatic cholestasis
G. Alpha-1-antitrypsin deficiency
H. Epstein–Barr virus infection
I. Hepatic vein thrombosis
J. Gallstones

The following patients are all jaundiced. Select the most likely aetiology from the list above.

1. A 32-year-old man presents to his GP after his wife had noticed that he had become jaundiced. He was not sure of the exact timescale but had definitely got worse over the last 2 weeks. He had been experiencing some right upper quadrant pain intermittently for some weeks. His only medication was mesalazine for a history of well-controlled ulcerative colitis. Bilirubin was 55 with elevated alkaline phosphatase of 980. The other liver enzymes are normal. ☐

2. A woman aged 35 years presents to A&E. She has had abdominal pain since the previous morning and had subsequently become noticeably jaundiced. Her abdomen was distended but there were no signs of chronic liver disease. She was normally fit and well and had a history of deep vein thrombosis 2 years ago for which she completed 6 months of warfarin therapy. There was no family history of liver disease although her mother had died suddenly in her 40s. ☐

3. A medical student had not been feeling well for several days. His tutor had noticed jaundiced sclera and arranged hospital admission. On examination, he has a temperature of 37.8 °C, tender submandibular lymphadenopathy, tender hepatomegaly and was clearly jaundiced. The splenic tip is just palpable. He had consumed 45 units of alcohol over the previous weekend. Alkaline phosphatase 500, ALT 85, GGT 90, bilirubin 43. Atypical lymphocytes are reported on a blood film. ☐

4. A man aged 64 years had become jaundiced over the preceding 2 weeks. This was not associated with pain or other gastrointestinal symptoms. On examination, he was thin without signs of chronic liver disease or hepatomegaly. Ultrasound demonstrated a dilated biliary tree and endoscopic retrograde cholangiopancreatography (ERCP) was suggested. ☐

5. A young man in his 20s attends his GP after noticing 'yellow eyes' for 2 days. Alkaline phosphatase 95, GGT 35, bilirubin 46, ALT 26, albumin 37. He was usually fit and well although he was just recovering from a heavy cold. There were no abnormal examination findings. ☐

8. THEME: Jaundice

A. Haemolysis
B. Gilbert's syndrome

9. THEME: Rectal bleeding

A. Diverticulosis
B. Haemorrhoids

C. Colonic carcinoma

D. Giardiasis

E. Diverticulitis

F. Angiodysplasia

G. Oesophageal variceal bleed

H. Ulcerative colitis

I. Amoebiasis

J. Cryptosporidiosis

The following patients all have a history of rectal bleeding. Select the most likely diagnosis from the list.

1. A 36-year-old man attends his GP as he is concerned about passing blood in his stools. This has occurred several times over the antecedent few weeks, with an associated history of 8–10 weeks of diarrhoea but no abdominal pain. He has no other significant medical history and is a non-smoker. There has been no recent travel abroad. Abdominal examination is interrupted by the patient having to rush to the toilet. Full blood count reveals a neutrophilia and a thrombocytosis. ☐

2. A woman aged 56 years is brought to A&E as an emergency after collapsing in the street. She has cold peripheries, hypotension, tachycardia and is barely conscious. A large volume of red blood has been passed PR, but there is no melaena evident. She has numerous spider naevi over her upper chest and back and has bilateral parotid swelling. ☐

3. A man aged 64 years presents to his GP with a history of several months of rectal bleeding. This has been intermittent, with small quantities of dark red blood sometimes mixed with the stool. His bowel habit has tended towards constipation. Abdominal examination reveals fullness in the left iliac fossa and rectal examination is normal. Full blood count and inflammatory markers are normal. He is referred for further investigation. ☐

4. A 47-year-old man has had rectal bleeding associated with diarrhoea for 3 days following a business trip to south-east Asia. He has also been very nauseated and has vomited twice. There is some lower abdominal tenderness but no other helpful clinical signs. He responds to empiric treatment with metronidazole while stool samples are analysed. ☐

5. A 54-year-old woman attends her GP with a history of dark red rectal bleeding. She has only noticed this over the last 10 days. The blood tends to be mixed with the stool. She has been opening her bowels twice a day for 2–3 months, whereas previously she was prone to constipation. She has lost 1 stone in weight over a 4-week period and attributes this to her thyroxine medication which started at this time. Full blood count demonstrates parameters consistent with iron deficiency. ☐

10. **THEME: Indigestion**

A. Reflux oesophagitis

B. Achalasia

C. Gastric carcinoma

D. Oesophageal spasm

E. Gastric ulceration

F. Acute gastritis

G. Myocardial infarction

H. Oesophageal candidiasis

I. Non-ulcer dyspepsia

J. Duodenal ulcer

The following patients all present with symptoms that they attribute to 'indigestion'. Try and establish what the most likely underlying diagnosis is, given the following information.

1. A man aged 42 years complains of indigestion. On further questioning, this has occurred intermittently over several weeks and consists of epigastric pain and discomfort. There are no effects with change in posture but it is worse at night. His weight has been steady. Full blood count is normal. ☐

2. A women aged 29 years attends her GP surgery complaining of persistent indigestion. She describes a sensation of epigastric fullness and early satiety. There have been no retrosternal symptoms or vomiting. Antacids are sometimes helpful. She does not take non-steroidal anti-inflammatory drugs (NSAIDs). Clinical examination is unrevealing. *Helicobacter pylori* serology is negative. ☐

3. A woman aged 34 years asks her GP for 'a tablet for indigestion'. Her symptoms have become particularly worse over the last 6 weeks. She describes a feeling of retrosternal burning that is related to posture. Antacids provide temporary relief. There has been no vomiting or melaena. There are no urinary symptoms although her period is late. Examination reveals a slightly overweight women, but no other significant findings. ☐

4. A man aged 63 years attends his GP one evening. He has had 'indigestion' since 05.00 hours. He describes it as a retrosternal burning or heaviness. He is normally fit and well, his only medication is bendrofluazide for hypertension with no NSAID use. He takes occasional antacids for postprandial dyspepsia but these have not helped today. On examination, he is sweating but there are no abnormal examination findings. ☐

5. A woman aged 44 years has had indigestion for several weeks. She describes epigastric discomfort and sometimes pain, precipitated by food. There are no retrosternal symptoms or a change in bowel habit. She is a smoker with no previous medical history. Routine FBC reveals Hb 10.8, WCC 9, Plt 440, MCV 74, MCH 22. ☐

He describes the diarrhoea as 'just water' with no visible blood and no abdominal pain. He feels dizzy on standing. Na 129, K 2.4, urea 26, Cr 204. He has a blood pressure of 110/70 mmHg and a pulse rate of 120 bpm. He is put on a drip and given tetracycline by the local hospital. ☐

3. A woman has just returned from the east coast of Africa. She started to feel unwell on the plane journey home. She was initially just vomiting, but has now developed bloody diarrhoea. On examination, there are areas of urticaria visible on her arms and legs and she is febrile. Sigmoidoscopy reveals mucosal ulceration. A rectal biopsy is taken. ☐

4. A man in his forties with known HIV infection has been feeling unwell for several weeks and attends his GP. He has lost weight and has been experiencing lower abdominal pain. His bowels are rather erratic and he attributes this to his medication. The right iliac fossa is tender and full blood count demonstrates a macrocytic anaemia. ☐

5. A middle-aged woman has been unwell for several days and she is brought to A&E by her husband. She has had a high temperature with sweats and has not been eating. Aside from a history of diabetes and diverticular disease, she has previously been well. There has been no foreign travel. On examination, a temperature of 38.4 °C is noted. She is tachycardic and the right lung base is dull to percussion. Alkaline phosphatase is 780 and bilirubin is 40. A Gram-negative organism is cultured in the blood. ☐

15. THEME: Adverse drug effects and toxicity on the gastrointestinal tract

A. Digoxin
B. Amiodarone
C. Flucloxacillin
D. Diclofenac
E. Atenolol
F. Low-dose aspirin
G. Ciprofloxacin
H. Metformin
I. Ferrous sulphate
J. Prednisolone
K. Fluconazole

The following patients have gastrointestinal/hepatobiliary problems related to prescribed medication. Identify the most likely culprit.

1. A 55-year-old man attends his GP with symptoms of lethargy, and feeling dizzy on standing. His only history is that of hypertension and hypercholesteraemia. On examination, his pulse rate is 98 bpm, blood pressure 122/72 mmHg. Abdomen soft, non-tender. Rectal examination: tarry stool. ☐

2. A 64-year-old woman is brought to A&E by her family. She is unwell, drowsy and dehydrated, and the only history is that of several days of diarrhoea. Na 135, K 6.3, urea 30, Cr 260, venous bicarbonate 10 (low), glucose 10. ☐

3. A man aged 78 years attends A&E with a history of nausea and vomiting. Bowels are normal and there is no haematemesis. He has felt dizzy intermittently. He has a 10-year history of diabetes mellitus. On examination, he has an irregular pulse and there are no signs of chronic liver disease or adverse abdominal findings. ☐

4. The boyfriend of a 27-year-old woman notices that her eyes look yellow and takes her to the GP. She is normally fit and well. She takes no regular medication but has recently been treated for a 'skin infection'. She also complains of vaginal thrush. She has a family history of hypercholesteraemia. On examination, she is jaundiced with no signs of chronic liver disease and no hepatomegaly. ☐

5. A 66-year-old retired engineer gives a history of several weeks of progressively becoming jaundiced. He had noticed this in the mirror. Otherwise, he felt quite well. His only history was that of a coronary angioplasty last year and a previous history of atrial fibrillation. On examination, his pulse was regular and there was no hepatomegaly or signs of chronic liver disease. ☐

16. THEME: Diarrhoea

A. *Campylobacter*
B. Whipple's disease
C. Coeliac disease
D. Irritable bowel syndrome
E. Small bowel bacterial overgrowth
F. Thyrotoxicosis
G. Collagenous colitis
H. Colon cancer
I. Ulcerative colitis
J. Pseudomembranous colitis

The following patients complain of diarrhoea. Identify which of these diagnoses is the most likely.

1. A 30-year-old man sees his GP complaining of bloody diarrhoea and cramping abdominal pain that had begun suddenly 1 week earlier. He describes headache, myalgia and fever which seem to be resolving. ☐

2. A 25-year-old woman is seen by her GP. She describes episodes over the last 10 years of loose stool associated with lower abdominal cramping discomfort and occasional bloating. She stopped smoking 6 months earlier and feels her symptoms are worse. She has recently noticed blood in her stools. ☐

3. A 25-year-old woman is seen by her GP. She describes episodes over the last 10 years of loose stool and passage of clear mucus associated

with lower abdominal cramping discomfort and occasional bloating.

4. A 70-year-old man is referred to the gastroenterology outpatient department. Five months earlier he noticed that he was opening his bowels more frequently, up to four or five times a day and was passing loose stool at times. He has lost some weight and he looks pale.

5. A 65-year-old man had a resection for a distal gastric cancer 15 years earlier. He has attended follow-up appointments and there has been no evidence of recurrence. He now complains of loose watery diarrhoea. Investigations reveal low vitamin B$_{12}$ levels and elevated folate levels.

17. THEME: Acute abdominal pain

A. Biliary colic
B. Appendicitis
C. Duodenal ulcer
D. Diverticulitis
E. Gastric ulcer
F. Crohn's disease
G. Cholecystitis
H. Hepatic vein thrombosis

The following patients develop acute abdominal pain. Identify the most likely cause of their pain.

1. A young woman on the oral contraceptive pill describes having had recurrent miscarriages in the past. She is admitted to hospital with abdominal pain, tender hepatomegaly and ascites.

2. A middle-aged woman is seen in A&E with upper abdominal pain. In the past she has had short-lived episodes of upper abdominal pain and is known to have gallstones. Now she complains of a 12-hour history of upper abdominal pain. Her temperature is elevated and blood tests reveal a leukocytosis.

3. A 27-year-old man is admitted with a 2-week history of epigastric pain. He describes a 'gnawing pain' that has woken him from sleep but has tended to be better during the day.

4. A 70-year-old woman describes colicky, left-sided abdominal pain associated with bloating and flatulence. She has a fever and a leukocytosis. There is mild left iliac fossa tenderness.

5. A young smoker complains of right iliac fossa pain. She feels generally unwell and nauseous. There is tenderness in the right iliac fossa and the impression of a fullness. These episodes have happened several times before.

18. THEME: Chronic abdominal pain

A. Chronic pancreatitis
B. Coeliac disease

C. Gastric cancer
D. Mesenteric ischaemia
E. Peptic ulcer disease
F. Crohn's disease
G. Irritable bowel syndrome
H. Colon cancer
I. Ulcerative colitis

Match the diagnosis to the following descriptions of patients with chronic abdominal pain.

1. A fifty year old man complains of intermittent episodes, each lasting 5–10 days, of central abdominal discomfort radiating to his back. He describes pale, offensive, bulky stools. Blood tests confirm vitamin B$_{12}$ deficiency, elevated MCV and raised GGT.

2. A 30-year-old woman has a 3-week history of epigastric discomfort exacerbated by food. Other than spraining her ankle a few weeks earlier, she is usually fit and well. She has noticed black stool at times.

3. A 25-year-old woman has a 3-year history of intermittent right iliac fossa pain accompanied by intermittent episodes of loose stool. She describes weight loss and fatigue. She attends the GP surgery as she is concerned that her symptoms are becoming progressively worse.

4. A 50-year-old man complains of a 3-month history of epigastric pain. He tries anatacids and then a proton pump inhibitor which only partially ease the discomfort. He complains of fatigue and weight loss. He is referred to the gastroenterology outpatient department by his GP.

5. A 45-year-old woman complains of bloating, lethargy and diffuse abdominal discomfort. This has been present for many years and she has been told in the past that she has irritable bowel syndrome. Her GP checks some blood tests and she is found to have folate deficiency and iron deficiency.

19. THEME: Dysphagia

A. Achalasia
B. Globus pharyngeus
C. Oesophageal cancer
D. Antral cancer
E. Schatzki ring
F. Candidiasis
G. Zenker's diverticulum
H. Oesophageal dysmotility
I. Scleroderma

The following patients have problems with swallowing. Identify the most likely diagnosis.

1. An elderly man has regurgitation and dysphagia. These symptoms have occurred intermittently for

over 1 year. His weight is stable and blood tests are normal. He feels otherwise well, but is concerned that his problems are not resolving. ☐

2. A 30-year-old woman complains of intermittent dysphagia to solids and liquids. She has no weight loss. A gastroscopy was normal. ☐

3. A 50-year-old man develops dysphagia to solid foods. On examination, he is found to have hyperkeratosis affecting his hands and feet. ☐

4. A 25-year-old woman sees her GP because she is being troubled by a recurrent sensation of a lump in the throat. Symptoms are worsened with repeated attempts to clear the lump by swallowing. She is worried that something may be intermittently sticking. However, her symptoms occur sporadically. In fact, on the day she comes to the gastroenterology unit for upper endoscopy, she is symptom free. ☐

5. A 50-year-old woman has had Reynaud's syndrome for many years. She has recently noticed a sensation of difficulty swallowing. On examination, she has some telangiectasia on her face. There is mild thickening of the skin on her fingers. ☐

20. THEME: Jaundice

A. Haemolysis
B. Alpha-1-antitrypsin (A-1-AT) deficiency
C. Primary biliary cirrhosis
D. Gallstones
E. Intra-hepatic cholestasis
F. Mirizzi's syndrome
G. Pancreatic cancer
H. Alcoholic hepatitis
I. Gilbert's syndrome

The following patients were admitted to hospital with jaundice. Match the clinical scenarios to the diagnosis.

1. A 50-year-old woman complains of right upper quadrant pain that is associated with light stool and dark urine. She attends the A&E department when her husband notices that she has become deeply jaundiced. ☐

2. A man in his 30s has emphysema. He has never smoked, but his lung disease is severe and limits his mobility. He has previously been noted to have mildly abnormal liver enzymes. He is admitted with a gradual onset of jaundice, which is not marked. ☐

3. A 60-year-old woman with a background of systemic lupus erythematosus (SLE) develops anaemia and jaundice. Her urine is normal in colour. Liver function tests show an isolated

elevated bilirubin. Other blood tests show an elevated lactate dehydrogenase level and reduced haptoglobin level. ☐

4. A young bodybuilder is admitted to hospital after his girlfriend notices that he has become jaundiced. He admits that this has happened before. He also describes pale stool and dark urine. ☐

5. A man in his early 30s is admitted with confusion and jaundice. His bilirubin level is $800 \, \mu mol/L$. There is little other history available. Examination reveals deep jaundice and some flapping tremor of the hands. He is confused. A liver biopsy report makes reference to the presence of 'Mallory's hyaline'. ☐

21. THEME: Rectal bleeding

A. Peptic ulcer
B. Diverticulosis
C. Ulcerative colitis
D. Acute ischaemic colitis
E. Haemorrhoids
F. Colon cancer
G. Angiodysplasia
H. Crohn's disease
I. Colonic polyps

The following patients have rectal bleeding. Identify the correct diagnosis from the list.

1. A man in his 30s had complained of vague abdominal pain for 2 weeks. He is rushed into hospital as an emergency. On arrival, his blood pressure is 70/40 mmHg, his pulse rate is 130 bpm and he has fresh blood rectally. ☐

2. A 76-year-old man has had symptoms for several years of occasional left iliac fossa pain and bloating. He is admitted with a brisk rectal bleed which resolves during his hospital stay. He is transfused 2 units of blood. One year later he remains well. ☐

3. A 30-year-old man has been treated for depression with amitriptyline. After a few weeks of treatment he attends his GP, as he has started to notice blood on the paper after opening his bowels. He is referred for a flexible sigmoidoscopy. ☐

4. A 60-year-old man is admitted with acute rectal blood loss. His past medical history is extensive and includes previous admissions with a heart attack and a stroke. He is awaiting angioplasty for peripheral vascular disease. The bleeding resolves over a period of days. He is investigated and discharged home. He is admitted 18 months later with subacute large bowel obstruction. ☐

5. A 60-year-old man is awaiting an aortic valve replacement. He is found to have iron-deficiency anaemia and therefore undergoes gastroscopy, sigmoidoscopy and barium enema. All of these investigations are normal. However, he continues to have recurrent iron-deficiency anaemia. He undergoes colonoscopy, which identifies the lesion causing his iron-deficiency anaemia. ☐

22. THEME: Vomiting

A. Gastric cancer
B. Digoxin toxicity
C. Rotavirus infection
D. *Salmonella* infection
E. *Shigella* infection
F. Peptic ulcer disease
G. Hypercalcaemia
I. Autonomic neuropathy
J. Intracranial neoplasm

Identify the cause of vomiting in the following patients.

1. An elderly lady is admitted after an episode of diarrhoea that lasted 1 week and has now resolved. However, she is now confused, vomiting and complains of an odd visual disturbance. She sees yellow-green haloes around lights. She has a past history of diabetes, ischaemic heart disease and atrial fibrillation. ☐

2. A 70-year-old woman with type 2 diabetes is admitted several times over the course of 1 year with episodes of vomiting. Each episode settles in hospital over a period of 7 days on average. Gastroscopy appears normal. Blood tests show only mild renal impairment. Her only other medical problems are mild diabetic retinopathy and a painless ulcer on her left foot. ☐

3. A cruise liner is quarantined at Southampton docks after an outbreak of vomiting among staff and passengers on board. The illness resolves within a few days in each passenger. After thorough cleaning, the cruise liner admits more passengers and continues on its journey. ☐

4. A 50-year-old lady has breast cancer. Over a period of a few weeks she complains of vomiting, constipation, fatigue and abdominal pain. During the course of her investigations, she is found to have renal stones. ☐

5. A 33-year-old man is referred to the gastroenterology outpatient department. He tends to wake in the morning with nausea, and a headache that eases as the day progresses. His symptoms have worsened in the last few weeks and he now vomits each morning. Blood tests are all normal and he undergoes gastroscopy and small bowel X-ray, which are normal. ☐

23. THEME: Infections of the gastrointestinal tract

A. Amoebiasis
B. Hepatitis A
C. *Helicobacter pylori*
D. Rotavirus
E. Giardiasis
F. Salmonellosis
G. Yersiniosis
H. *Clostridium difficile*

Identify the infective aetiology in the following scenarios.

1. A woman returns from holiday in St Petersburg. She develops diarrhoea, fever and abdominal discomfort. All of her fellow travel companions suffer the same symptoms. She drops off a stool culture which is received and processed in the pathology department the following day. It is negative. ☐

2. A 25-year-old man is admitted a couple of days after having eaten undercooked pork at a barbecue. He has fever, diarrhoea and right-sided iliac fossa pain. Clinically, his symptoms seem very much like those of appendicitis. ☐

3. A woman sees her GP complaining of diarrhoea, abdominal cramps and vomiting. Her family have all had the same problem. She ate undercooked poultry the day before. ☐

4. A traveller returns from her journey to a developing country with a mild flu-like illness. She develops jaundice which resolves over the following 6 weeks. She is a smoker. However, during this time, she notices that her craving for cigarettes is markedly diminished. ☐

5. A 70-year-old woman attends the A&E department after developing jaundice. She has been unwell for some weeks with malaise and anorexia. She is febrile and, on examination, is found to have tender hepatomegaly. When asked about foreign travel, she admits that although she has not left the UK for some years, she used to live and work in the Tropics. ☐

d. True Alkaline phosphatase, gamma-glutamyl transferase and bilirubin are commonly elevated.

e. False This can be helpful in assessing dilated bile ducts or detecting ovarian cysts.

11. a. True This is often relevant (and may be painless)—do not forget low-dose aspirin.

b. True Typically of gastric ulcers (may relieve pain of duodenal ulceration).

c. False Altered blood, manifest as melaena, is sometimes a feature.

d. False This suggests a gastrointestinal malignancy and does not occur with peptic ulcers.

e. True This can be a feature—particularly of duodenal ulcers.

12. a. False The amylase is frequently normal, in contradistinction to acute pancreatitis.

b. False Some features may be revealing but it is infrequently of diagnostic help.

c. True A high platelet count can also be seen with chronic blood loss.

d. True Particularly if the terminal ileum is involved.

e. False This occurs with vitamin B_{12} and folate deficiency—microcytosis is found in this context.

13. a. False Nephrotic syndrome is a hypoalbuminaemic state leading to ascites with a low protein content.

b. False Cytological examination may reveal a neoplastic process, but this is not excluded by the absence of malignant cells.

c. True ECG changes of cardiac failure or constrictive pericarditis may be evident.

d. True This is the diagnostic modality of choice for the detection of ascites.

e. True The appearance may be suggestive of constrictive pericarditis or cardiac failure.

14. a. False Patients often over- or underestimate the extent of their weight loss.

b. True A hypermetabolic state is thought to be the underlying mechanism, although anorexia may contribute.

c. True This combination of symptoms would be typical for a hyperthyroid state.

d. True As would a low urea and low albumin.

e. False Corticosteroids tend to induce weight gain— hypoadrenalism can cause weight loss.

15. a. False This would be unusual, although they can contribute toward peptic ulceration.

b. True Particularly if drug levels are in the toxic range.

c. True Many antibiotics are culprits. Metronidazole commonly does.

d. False Non-steroidal anti-inflammatory drugs (NSAIDs) tend to cause dyspepsia/reflux symptoms rather than vomiting per se.

e. True All opiates, including codeine, frequently cause vomiting.

16. a. True Usually when the blood glucose gets very high.

b. False Different symptoms: sweating/hunger/ tremor/altered consciousness/fits.

c. True Also constipation, abdominal pain, thirst and polyuria.

d. False Does not usually lead to vomiting.

e. True Particularly in chronic renal failure.

17. a. False Melaena should always follow a true haematemesis.

b. True This indicates the patient is anticoagulated and subsequently at higher risk of a significant bleed.

c. True Suggests intravascular depletion and is often evident before systolic pressure falls.

d. True Until haemodilution of intravascular volume occurs.

e. False This history would more likely indicate a Mallory–Weiss tear.

18. a. False A low urea can be seen with liver disease—a high urea indicates a significant bleed.

b. False Coagulopathy can indicate impairment of hepatic synthetic function.

c. True A reactive phenomenon of the bone marrow.

d. True Hypersplenism consequent upon portal hypertension is associated with varices.

e. False The national standard is that endoscopy should follow all gastrointestinal bleeds (although there is clearly a spectrum of urgency).

19. a. True Elderly patients have a poorer outcome from acute bleeding.

b. False Although aetiologically relevant, NSAIDs do not influence outcome.

c. True These patients are less able to cope with the haemodynamic stresses.

d. True Hypovolaemia results in 'pre-renal' deterioration in function.

e. True Can reflect preceding blood loss.

20. a. False Constipation with opiates is the norm.

b. True Antibiotics such as the penicillins and cephalosporins are often culprits.

c. True (Used in gout.) Is often dose dependent.

d. False Not a well recognized side effect of this drug class.

e. False This antibiotic is used to treat diarrhoea associated with pseudomembranous colitis (*Clostridium difficile* overgrowth).

21. a. True Reflects mucosal inflammation.

b. False Affects small intestine, watery, non-bloody diarrhoea.

c. True Can present a long time following radiotherapy.

d. False The presence of blood indicates more significant pathology.

e. False Causes diarrhoea, but not bloody.

22. a. False   A normocytic or microcytic picture is seen reflecting chronic disease or iron deficiency respectively.

b. True   Urinary 5-HIAA, a serotonin metabolite, is elevated in carcinoid syndrome.

c. False   Aetiology is usually viral, although bacterial infection must be excluded.

d. True   May occur despite iron deficiency—ferritin acts as an inflammatory protein.

e. False   Not frequently—toxic dilatation/faecal impaction or pancreatic calcification may be seen.

23. a. True.

b. True.

c. True.

d. False.

e. True.

Steatorrhoea is seen with malabsorption, either due to (proximal) small intestinal disease or pancreatic insufficiency.

24. a. True   Commonly implicated.

b. False   Although usually in the immunocompromised.

c. True   Often as a consequence of poor food hygiene.

d. False   Rarely causes diarrhoea.

e. False   Often via contaminated water, severe in patients with AIDS.

25. a. True   Reflects dehydration; often disproportionately elevated to the serum creatinine.

b. False   (Unless acute renal failure has resulted!) Hypokalaemia reflects excess gut loss.

c. True   Often mirrors the potassium level.

d. False   This tends to cause constipation.

e. True   Poor diabetic control can lead to autonomic neuropathy.

26. a. False   Bright red blood is more typical of haemorrhoids.

b. False   This pattern more often represents high rectal lesions such as carcinoma, angiodysplasia or inflamed diverticula.

c. True   You would expect to find increased anal tone and pain on rectal examination.

d. False   This would be a more characteristic feature of diverticulitis.

e. False   Blood loss from 'simple' anorectal conditions is rarely severe enough to result in anaemia—carcinoma, inflammatory bowel disease and angiodysplasia are more likely.

27. a. True   Further investigation is only required in equivocal cases.

b. True   And if there is a high level of clinical suspicion.

c. False   Rigid sigmoidoscopy is limited to 15–20 cm range.

d. False   Proctoscopy is rarely tolerated in patients with anal fissure.

e. False   Haemorrhoids are common incidental findings and not always the culprit lesion.

28. a. False   Pale conjunctivae correlate very poorly with haemoglobin concentration.

b. True   Particularly the mean cell volume (MCV).

c. True   To exclude oesophagitis, gastric ulcer/ erosions or carcinoma.

d. False   In isolation, this finding is an insufficient explanation.

e. False   This is a common cause in the UK and Ireland.

29. a. False   These drugs have an *anti-folate* action.

b. True   Reticulocytes are large red cell precursors, seen in a marrow response to bleeding or haemolysis.

c. False   Caecal carcinoma causes a microcytic, iron-deficient picture.

d. False   This test helps differentiate between the different causes of vitamin B_{12} deficiency.

e. True   On its own, or in association with pernicious anaemia.

30. a. False   This suggests anaemia of chronic disease. Total iron-binding capacity should be raised in iron deficiency.

b. True   As a consequence of gastric erosions.

c. True   Established from the context and history.

d. True   Coeliac disease can lead to either iron or folate deficiency, or both.

e. False   These are seen in vitamin B_{12}/folate deficiency.

31. a. False   Usually detectable in sclera at levels greater than 40 µmol/L.

b. False   A rapid onset is more likely to be an infective cause.

c. False   This contravenes Courvoisier's law.

d. True   This differentiates obstructive jaundice from other causes.

e. False   Prothrombin time is a better indicator of synthetic function.

32. a. True   Typically a cholestatic picture.

b. True   In excess of therapeutic dose.

c. False   Uncommon.

d. False   Predominantly nephrotoxic.

e. True   Such as isoniazid and rifampicin.

33. a. True   Infections such as cytomegalovirus, Epstein–Barr virus or toxoplasmosis.

b. True   Chronic liver disease/cirrhosis (Budd–Chiari if acute).

c. True   Wilson's disease also affects the basal ganglia.

d. True   Another sign of chronic liver disease.

e. True   Cardiac failure can lead to hepatic congestion.

34. a. False   Levels of alanine aminotransferase (ALT) do not correlate well with liver *function*.

b. False   Alkaline phosphatase has non-hepatic sources: bone/placenta/small intestine

c. True   Raised gamma-glutamyl transferase (GGT) in isolation is very suggestive of this.

d. False   A typical metastatic picture is elevated ALT and GGT.

e. True   Enquire about night sweats, weight loss and skin rash.

94. a. False   This is bound to albumin—*conjugated* bilirubin is water soluble.
    b. False   Via the *portal* vein.
    c. False   About 15% have a cholecystectomy for symptoms attributable to gallstones.
    d. False   Only approximately 10% are seen on plain X-ray.
    e. True   Cholesterol stones (reduced bile salts in the liver).

95. a. True   Obstruction/swelling of the ampulla of Vater caused by gallstones.
    b. False   Not causally associated.
    c. True   Infection spreading into intra-hepatic ducts.
    d. False   An entirely distinct pathology.
    e. True   Can present with swinging fever and septi-caemia.

96. a. True   Sphincter of Oddi and gastric acid help maintain this.
    b. True   *Escherichia coli* being the commonest organism implicated.
    c. True   With elevation of alkaline phosphatase and bilirubin—transaminase elevation usually mild.
    d. False   Frequently positive—90% if repeated cultures are taken.
    e. True   Especially if a stent is inserted.

97. a. True   Massive pooling of intravascular fluid around the pancreas—'third space losses'.
    b. False   Not a typical presentation.
    c. True   Very common, severe and often radiates to the back.

    d. True   Almost invariable.
    e. True   Particularly in severe cases and if adult respiratory distress syndrome is a complication.

98. a. False   A potential complication (*hyper*calcaemia is a cause).
    b. False   A potential complication due to loss of endocrine function.
    c. True   Particularly at high doses.
    d. True   A common cause.
    e. False   Scorpion bite!

99. a. True   Blood cultures should always be performed at presentation.
    b. True   Oral hypoglycaemics/insulin may be required short or long term.
    c. True   Can be life threatening; perform a coagulation screen, fibrinogen and D-dimers.
    d. True   Paralytic ileus is commonly seen.
    e. True   Usually as a result of hypovolaemia ± sepsis ± disseminated intravascular coagulation.

100. a. False   Usually normal in chronic pancreatitis.
    b. True   Pancreatic duct dilatation/distortion may be seen.
    c. False   Can be seen in up to 50% of moderate to severe cases.
    d. True   A paraneoplastic skin manifestation.
    e. False   Late—often with hepatomegaly and liver metastases.

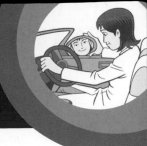

1. The pattern of enzyme abnormality (and the history of itching) suggests a cholestatic process. The single most useful investigation is a hepatobiliary ultrasound to assess the biliary tree. If the bile ducts are not dilated, all hepatic causes (especially those causing intra-hepatic cholestasis) should be considered. In a middle-aged woman, primary biliary cirrhosis is a distinct possibility (check anti-mito-chondrial (M2) antibodies). She may have been given co-amoxiclav for a respiratory infection, which would be a prime suspect as an aetiological agent in cholestatic jaundice.

2. There is clinical evidence of shock. This could be as a result of sepsis, intravascular volume loss, or both. You should consider acute appendicitis with perforation or abscess, Crohn's disease, ectopic pregnancy, ruptured ovarian cyst and acute pyelonephritis. Investigations should include a pregnancy test, ultrasound scan, mid-stream urine for culture and possibly further imaging with a small bowel enema.

3. A low ferritin would confirm iron deficiency, although a normal or high ferritin should be interpreted with caution, as it is an acute phase (inflammatory) protein. Low serum iron and high iron-binding capacity are also supportive of iron deficiency. The finding of a duodenal ulcer should prompt acid suppression and *Helicobacter pylori* eradication, if appropriate, but should not necessarily be accepted as the cause of the iron deficiency. The lower gastrointestinal tract should be investigated with colonoscopy or barium enema. Check whether duodenal biopsies were taken at the time of the initial endoscopy (exclude coeliac disease).

4. Ulcerative colitis (UC) is more likely to present with bloody diarrhoea than Crohn's disease. Mouth ulcers are common in Crohn's as the entire length of the gastrointestinal tract can be affected. It characteristically affects the terminal ileum or small intestine, which are usually unaffected by UC. The rectum is almost always inflamed in UC and usually spared in Crohn's. Ulcerative colitis causes superficial ulceration, whereas Crohn's is a transmural disease causing deep ulcers. Histology may demonstrate crypt abscesses in UC and granulomata in Crohn's. Crohn's is more common in smokers. Perianal disease, with abscesses or fistulae, is more common in Crohn's disease.

5. Low PO_2, high lactate dehydrogenase, high white cell count, high glucose, low calcium, high urea, low albumin and high aspartate aminotransferase are poor prognostic signs in acute pancreatitis. Initial management should include: oxygen if hypoxic (and perform a chest X-ray); adequate venous access and fluid resuscitation; a urinary catheter is often required; consider a central venous line (particularly if there is existing cardiac impairment); adequate analgesia and antiemetics; blood cultures and broad-spectrum antibiotics if there is evidence of sepsis. A coagulation screen should be performed to look for evidence of disseminated intravascular coagulation. Always get senior help.

6. The human leucocyte antigen B_{27} is associated with a group of inflammatory conditions known as the spondylarthritides because a prominent feature is an inflammatory arthritis, usually of the spine. They include ankylosing spondylitis, psoriatic arthropathy and Reiter' disease (an asymmetrical arthritis with urethritis, uveitis and, occasionally, colitis). All of these conditions are associated with ulcerative colitis. It is postulated to be an immune phenomenon related to *Salmonella* or *Chlamydia* infection.

7. Characteristically, a low albumin, low calcium and phosphate (vitamin D deficiency) are seen. Urea may also be low, although does not correlate well with nutritional state. Prothrombin time may be prolonged if vitamin K deficiency has occurred. Anaemia may be seen: microcytic if iron-deficient, macrocytic if B_{12}/folate deficient, or normocytic if combined haematinic deficiency exists. Normocytic anaemia may also reflect a 'chronic disease/inflammatory process'. Abnormal liver function tests may give aetiological clues. Inflammatory markers such as C-reactive protein may also help in this respect. Causes of malabsorption in a man this age include coeliac disease, Crohn's disease, chronic pancreatitis, bacterial overgrowth and infections such as giardiasis. Hyperthyroidism and diabetes mellitus should be excluded.

8. This man presents with features suggestive of cholangitis. It is likely that the endoprosthesis has become occluded and the bilary tree has ascending infection. Blood cultures may reveal the causative organism, most commonly *Escherichia coli*. Broad-spectrum antibiotics to cover Gram-negative and anaerobic organisms should be used in the first instance. Liver function tests will suggest cholestasis; a neutrophilia may be seen with elevated inflammatory markers. He should undergo an urgent biliary ultrasound and the stent should subsequently be removed and replaced.

9. Endoscopy with biopsy for histology, culture or a 'clo (urease) test' can be employed at the time of biopsy. Alternative, non-invasive approaches would include a serological (IgG) test that indicates past infection, but will remain positive following eradication. A urease breath test can also be employed (see Chs 15 and 24). Triple therapy

may include amoxicillin, metronidazole and a proton pump inhibitor such as lansoprazole. Alcohol should be avoided in combination with metronidazole, as extremely unpleasant reactions would occur (nausea, vomiting and flushing). This occurs because metronidazole inhibits the enzyme acetaldehyde dehydrogenase, resulting in accumulation of the offending metabolite.

10. You need to establish the exact timing of the overdose and whether or not any other prescription or illicit drugs were consumed. A history of alcohol excess or underlying liver or renal impairment is also relevant. A psychiatric history should also be taken to assess suicidal intent. Serum paracetamol levels are plotted on a Prescott nomogram and correlated to time post ingestion to establish the need for treatment, but the timing may be difficult if the history is unreliable. It is usually safer to treat if any doubt remains. A low pH, high creatinine and prolonged prothrombin time have been shown to adversely affect outcome.

11. This is a common age for Gilbert' syndrome to present, and is the most likely explanation for the isolated hyperbilirubinaemia in this context. The normal gamma-glutamyl transferase implies that the alkaline phosphatase may be from a non-hepatic source (isoenzymes of alkaline phosphatase can be measured to determine the organ of origin). In this case, the elevated alkaline phosphatase reflects actively growing bones. Red cell haemolysis should be considered, and a reticulocyte count performed. The mechanism of the hyperbilirubinaemia involves a reduction in enzyme activity (glucuronosyl transferase or UGT-1), and thus a reduction in conjugation of bilirubin.

12. Pernicious anaemia should be considered. Autoantibodies to parietal cells are found in 90%; there may also be antibodies to intrinsic factor. A Schilling test (see Ch. 24) may be appropriate to differentiate between lack of intrinsic factor and terminal ileal disease (e.g. Crohn's or tuberculosis). Malabsorption due to small intestinal disease should be considered, particularly in younger patients with vitamin B_{12} deficiency. Other causes of a macrocytosis include alcohol excess, folate deficiency, hypothyroidism, myelodysplasia, hyperlipidaemia and chronic hypoxia. A reticulocytosis can also manifest as a 'spurious' macrocytosis.

13. This patient has clear evidence of hepatic encephalopathy. Convulsions and coma are seen in severe cases, or signs may be as subtle as constructional apraxia or mild irritability. Acute onset usually has a precipitating factor which can be potentially reversible; for example, bleeding, infection (bacterial or fungal) or drugs. Grade of encephalopathy is one parameter used to assess the functional capacity of the liver. The others are raised bilirubin, lowered albumin, ascites and coagulopathy (prolonged prothrombin time).

14. Features indicating severity in ulcerative colitis include: stool frequency of less than eight times per day with blood, abdominal pain and tenderness; fever >37.5 °C; tachycardia >100 bpm; C-reactive protein >20; erythrocyte sedimentation rate >35; haemoglobin <10; albumin <30. Abdominal pain is often an ominous sign and an abdominal radiograph should be performed to look for evidence of toxic megacolon. The history of 'shivers' may indicate superimposed sepsis (bacteraemia resulting from damaged colonic mucosa). Blood and stool cultures should be performed and broad-spectrum antibiotics initiated if suspicion exists. Aggressive fluid resuscitation is often required. A stool chart, strict fluid balance charting and a daily weight are imperative. Corticosteroids are usually given during an acute attack to induce remission. Further immunosuppression and surgical intervention may be required.

15. Liver biopsy is the definitive test for diagnosis and at the same time assesses the extent of liver damage. The hepatic iron index is of particular value (see Ch. 18). Ferritin is an 'acute phase' protein and can be (misleadingly) elevated in infections or inflammatory states. Other manifestations of haemochromatosis include: hypogonadotrophic hypogonadism (pituitary); pigmentation of skin; porphyria cutanea tarda (skin photosensitivity); arthritis of the small joints of the hand; chondrocalcinosis (knees); cardiomyopathy; and diabetes mellitus (pancreatic damage). The patient is also at risk of hepatoma and the other complications of cirrhosis.

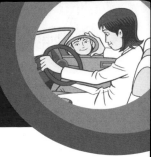

1. THEME: Haematemesis and melaena

1. E This lady is taking non-steroidal anti-inflammatory drugs (NSAIDs) for her arthritis; these ulcers are often painless and may present with acute bleeds.
2. B Large variceal bleed in a patient with known cirrhosis and consequent portal hypertension. These patients sometimes have thrombocytopenia because of liver disease/splenomegaly/alcohol toxicity, thus increasing the bleeding risk.
3. C A typical history of Mallory–Weiss. Of note, the streaks of blood only appeared in later episodes of vomiting.
4. D Significant weight loss has occurred and the indices are those of iron deficiency. Gastric carcinoma is commoner with advancing age. Note the high platelet count, consistent with chronic bleeding.
5. I Pain from duodenal ulceration is classically worse with hunger and relieved with food. Ninety-five per cent of duodenal ulcers are associated with *Helicobacter pylori* infection.

2. THEME: Diarrhoea

1. B Coeliac disease is particularly common in the west of Ireland and has a second peak of incidence in this age group. It commonly causes an iron-deficiency picture through malabsorption.
2. D Giardiasis is common in the tropics and can cause malabsorption. Repeat stool culture is often necessary to identify cysts. *Campylobacter* is less likely because of the significant weight loss and no blood in the stool.
3. C *Clostridium difficile* toxin-associated diarrhoea often occurs following recent antibiotic treatment (e.g. penicillins, cephalosporins, clindamycin).
4. A Terminal ileum involvement is common in Crohn's, producing right iliac fossa pain. 'Anaemia of chronic disease' with elevated inflammatory markers can occur.
5. H The clues to thyrotoxicosis here are weight loss with a good appetite, anxiety and irregular pulse (atrial fibrillation).

3. THEME: Acute abdominal pain

1. J Acute bowel infarction caused by mesenteric thrombosis. He has 'vascular' risk factors of smoking and, notably, atrial fibrillation. A lactic (metabolic) acidosis is very common. The mortality is high.
2. C A jaundiced middle-aged woman with right upper quadrant pain. The diagnosis is supported by the pattern of liver enzymes and *Escherichia coli* septicaemia.
3. F Gallstones are a common cause of acute pancreatitis in the UK. She has evidence of shock and is likely to be tachypnoeic as a result of a metabolic acidosis, or may be developing acute respiratory distress syndrome.
4. H He is dehydrated (polyuria) clinically and biochemically and has a very low venous bicarbonate (metabolic acidosis). The hyperkalaemia and breathlessness are a result of the acidosis. Never forget glucose!
5. I The differential, of course, includes appendicitis. However, the history is short and she has evidence of significant intravascular volume loss.

4. THEME: Chronic abdominal pain

1. G Pancreatic carcinoma is often associated with significant weight loss and the pain is persistent and often severe.
2. I There is evidence of inflammation and the site of pain suggests a biliary origin. Ultrasound may demonstrate a shrunken gall bladder with evidence of chronic inflammation.
3. F A typical history for irritable bowel syndrome, alternating bowel habit with a rather vague history of abdominal pain. The negative findings mentioned and normal inflammatory markers lead one away from an inflammatory aetiology.
4. B This man has probably been seeing a neurologist for transient ischaemic attacks. The timing of the pain coincides with a few hours after the evening meal. A degree of malabsorption can occur with mesenteric ischaemia.
5. H This man probably has a history of coeliac disease although the recent story of soaking night sweats, abdominal pain, weight loss and elevated LDH are suggestive of non-Hodgkin's lymphoma. This may well be an enteropathy-associated T lymphoma (EATL).

5. THEME: Anaemia

1. F The operation was likely to be a partial gastrectomy and the resulting anatomy has encouraged bacterial overgrowth. Clinical and biochemical features of malabsorption are typical and a high folate is the consequence of bacterial metabolism.
2. D The indices indicate iron deficiency with the slightly high platelet count suggestive of chronic bleeding. No lesion was identified at upper or lower gastrointestinal investigation but the bleeding evidently was recurrent. A radioisotope labelled red cell scan is sometimes helpful if bleeding is active.

numerous guises (see Ch. 15). 'Mechanical' problems such as afferent loop syndrome (rare) can be mentioned, as should the increased risk of carcinoma that is observed.

9. Carcinoid syndrome fits with the clinical picture and ultrasound findings. Clinical features can also include bronchospasm and cardiac lesions (seen in 50%). The tumour originates from amine precursor uptake and decarboxylation (APUD) cells. Common primary sites include the appendix, terminal ileum and rectum. The hormones most commonly secreted are serotonin (5-HT), bradykinin and histamines. The syndrome is only seen in those with liver metastases. Diagnosis can be supported by detecting the major metabolite of serotonin in the urine or by radioisotope techniques. See Ch. 16 for further details.

10. The history is strongly suggestive of achalasia. Presentation in childhood is unusual. This rare condition also commonly presents with chest pain as a result of oesophageal spasm. Dysphagia can also be overcome by drinking large quantities of fluid (with the risk of aspiration). Endoscopy can be useful to obtain biopsy, although can sometimes miss the oesophageal narrowing. An endoscopic ultrasound is helpful in excluding malignant infiltration, should this be suspected. Specific treatment can include balloon dilatation or surgical division of muscle fibres. Calcium channel blockers can reduce oesophageal spasm and can be useful in elderly patients who may not be suitable for invasive procedures. The risk of carcinoma is significantly higher and reflux oesophagitis is common following treatment.

Index

A

abdomen
  auscultation 193
  palpation 192–3
  percussion 193
  scars 193, 194
abdominal aortic aneurysm
  abdominal pain 16
  chest X-ray 18
  symptoms 17
abdominal distension 27–30
  afferent loop syndrome 87
  bowel habit 28
  examination 28
  investigation 28–30
    cardiac investigation 30
    radiology 29
  irritable bowel syndrome 107
  with jaundice 55
  onset of symptoms 27
  pain
    acute 17
    chronic 22
  patient history 27–8
  patterns of 29
abdominal examination
  general examination 192–3, 194
  weight loss 32
abdominal mass
  abdominal pain, chronic 23
  general examination 193, 195
abdominal pain 192
  acute 15–20
    character of pain 16
    differential diagnosis 15
    distension 17
    examination 16–17
    family history 16
    guarding and rebound tenderness 16–17
    hernial orifices and male genitalia 17
    internal examination 17
    investigations 17–20
      biochemistry 17–18
      endoscopy 20
      full blood count 17
      radiology 18–19
      surgery 20
    medical history 16

    patient history 15–16
    pulsation 17
    radiation of pain 16
    relieving and exacerbating factors 16
    site of pain 15
    site of tenderness 17
  afferent loop syndrome 87
  amoebiasis 124
  bacterial infection of the colon 123
  chronic 21–5
    associated features 22
    character 21–2
    differential diagnosis 21
    exacerbating and relieving
      factors 22
    examination 22–3
    investigations 23–5
      biochemistry 23
      endoscopy 24
      full blood count 23
      radiology 23–4
      surgery 25
    patient history 21–2
    site and radiation of pain 21
  coeliac disease 91
  colorectal carcinoma 118
  Crohn's disease 21
  cryptosporidiosis 124
  drug toxicity 157
  gastric carcinoma 84
  gastric polyps 81
  hydatid disease 161
  irritable bowel syndrome 107
  with jaundice 55
  Ménétrièr's disease 83
  pancreatic carcinoma 178
  primary sclerosing cholangitis 144
  pseudocysts 177
  pyogenic abscess 159
  schistosomiasis 162
  ulcerative colitis 110
abdominal ultrasound 220
  abdominal distension 29
  abdominal pain, chronic 23
  colorectal carcinoma 118
  jaundice 55–6
  tuberculosis 101
  weight loss 33
abdominal wall discolouration 173

273

loop diuretics, cirrhosis 152
lower limb examination 191, 192
lower oesophageal sphincter (LOS) 63, 64, 71
lower oesophageal web 12, 70, 71
Lundh test 209
lung transplant 178
lupus erythematosus (LE) cells 146
lymph node biopsy 102
lymphadenopathy
    bilateral hilar 146
    brucellosis 137
    intra-abdominal 23
    rectal bleeding 47
    toxoplasmosis 136
    with weight loss 32
lymphocytes, toxoplasmosis 137
lymphocytic colitis 114
Lynch syndrome type I 118

M

macrocytic anaemia 45, 51
macrocytosis 59, 149, 201
macronodular cirrhosis 150
maculopapular rash
    hepatitis B 131
    toxoplasmosis 137
magnesium 204
magnetic resonance cholangiography
    gallstones 167
    jaundice 56
magnetic resonance cholangiopancreatography
        (MRCP)
    cholangiocarcinoma 170
    primary sclerosing cholangitis 145
magnetic resonance imaging (MRI) scan 221
    abdominal distension 29
    anal fistula 122
    colorectal carcinoma 118
    Crohn's disease 96
    hepatocellular carcinoma 156
malabsorption 33, 50
    bacterial overgrowth 100
    coeliac disease 92
    Crohn's disease 94
    cystic fibrosis 178
    diarrhoea 44
    fat 209
    following gastric surgery 89
    intestinal lymphoma 98
    pancreatitis, chronic 176
    steatorrhoea 44
malaise
    Epstein–Barr virus 136
    fascioliasis 162
    gall bladder carcinoma 170

hepatitis A 130
hepatitis C 134
pyogenic abscess 159
schistosomiasis 162
male genitalia examination in acute abdominal pain 17
malignancy
    diarrhoea 44
    vomiting 37
    see also tumour(s); specific malignancy
Mallory bodies 148
Mallory–Weiss tear 40
malnutrition 33
    coeliac disease 92–3
    gastroparesis 85
maltoma 78
mania, facial signs of 189
manometry
    anorectal 210
    bile duct 219
    megacolon 109
    oesophageal 7, 63, 210, 211
mean cell volume (MCV) 202
mebendazole
    hookworm infection 104
    roundworm infection 105
    threadworm infection 126
    whipworm infection 125
Meckel's diverticulum 52
meconium ileus 178
medical clerking, writing up 197–200
    continuity 198
    formulating a differential diagnosis 197
    illustration 197
    investigation 198
    purpose 197
    sample 198–200
    structure 197
megacolon 45–6, 109
    toxic 110, 111–12, 113
melaena 39–41
    anaemia 50
    causes of 39
    variceal bleeding 152
Ménétrièr's disease 83
meningitis 36, 37
menstruation
    abdominal distension 27
    abdominal pain, chronic 22
    as a cause of anaemia 49
6-mercaptopurine, Crohn's disease 96
mesalazine
    Crohn's disease 96
    microscopic colitis 115
    ulcerative colitis 112–13, 114
mesenteric adenitis 102